Internal Fitness

Scott Basto, DC

Legal Disclaimers and Notices

I would like to dedicate this book to the memory of two great pioneers in the field of alternative health care. They were inspirational teachers and mentors.

Major Bertrand De Jarnette, D.C. developed Chiropractic Manipulative Reflex Technique as part of Sacro Occipital Technique.

George J. Goodheart, D.C. advanced the development of Applied Kinesiology.

Table of Contents

About the Author

A graduate of the University of Virginia and Palmer College of Chiropractic, Dr. Basto has practiced in the Healing Arts for 30 years with private practices in Florida, Hawaii and Colorado. He has studied with doctors, nutritionists and biochemists throughout the United States and Europe. The systems and procedures in this book are based on these studies and 30 years of clinical trials with patients.

Taking Care of Yourself

In the early 1970's, I had the good fortune to be in the Peace Corps. My host country was the Western Caroline Islands. As part of my language training program, I spent several days in the jungle with one of the islanders. I learned more than a new language on the trip. Just observing Atoon, as he functioned in his native environment, was an enlightening experience.

Atoon slithered through the overgrown jungle silently, hardly disturbing plant or animal. He knew where to drink the water, and where not to drink the water. He could spear several fish for dinner in five minutes, using just a sharpened wooden stick, while standing in knee deep water. He cooked them whole over the glow of a dried coconut husk that he set afire and held in his hand. These were all the wonderful aspects of life that I expected to see in this primitive culture.

What surprised me was the way Atoon used his environment for health maintenance beyond just the expected food, clothing and shelter. At one point, he cut himself rather deeply on a stiff sharp-edged plant leaf. I was quite concerned because it looked like it was going to be a real "bleeder", and we were carrying no first aid provisions. My friend was at home in the jungle, of course, and calmly looked around until he found the plant that he knew he needed. He then pulled off a leaf, and pressed it onto his wound. The bleeding stopped immediately, and the wound was sealed. No further treatment was required.

When it came time to eat our fish, Atoon again searched for the right plant, stripped all the leaves off one branch, and gave half of them to me. Then he knelt down by a clear stream, wet the leaves, and rubbed them together in the palms of his hands. Instantly, thick white suds were produced as the leaves soaped away the day's dirt. My entire stay in those Pacific Islands was an ongoing reminder of how wonderfully competent nature can be in taking care of us, if we make the effort to care for ourselves.

The islanders around me ate fresh fish, fresh fruit and rice, and chewed betel nut. There was no dentist, doctor or hospital on the island. The islanders were rarely sick and had no tooth decay.

Simple, natural diets, such as this, are difficult to incorporate into a busy lifestyle, today, so you must find alternate ways to stay healthy. Fortunately, the human body is very adaptive. It is continuously adjusting and repairing to compensate for internal and external environments. Often we block, with lifestyle, the body's efforts to repair. *Internal Fitness* explains how you can restore your body's pathway to repair and rejuvenation. Throughout 30 years of practice, I have used the procedures in this book to help my patients overcome countless health problems.

My objective in writing *Internal Fitness* was to create a tool with which you can improve your health. Use this book to realize better health regardless of your present condition. The information on the following pages will assist you in this endeavor whether you are a couch potato or a tri-athlete.

With *Internal Fitness*, I have presented a program in which you use no equipment other than your own hands to elevate your state of health. You need no special clothing, no special room, no trainer, and no ideal weather conditions. You will use the Complaint Chart for evaluation, then, complete a Reflex Scan to identify problem areas. After this, the procedures take only minutes a day. You should, therefore, be able to incorporate this program without altering your lifestyle. I frequently recommend that the procedural segment of the program be performed in bed after retiring for the evening. Once you have memorized the procedure, you can perform it just before you go to sleep. In this way, you will not have to take time away from your busy schedule. These strengthening procedures use neurologic reflexes to trigger the repair and recovery mechanisms of your body.

If you wish to strengthen your external musculature, you feed the muscle tissue a proper combination of amino acids, vitamins and minerals. You then exercise to stimulate the utilization of that nutrition for the purpose of increasing the size of each muscle belly that is being worked. You are not actually adding muscle, but rather, increasing the size and strength of the muscle tissue already there.

With *Internal Fitness*, you are going to learn how to strengthen your internal systems. Instead of nutrition and exercise, the mechanism will be nutrition and reflex stimulation. With this combination, remarkable repair and rejuvenation is possible. *Internal Fitness* gives you the capability of developing a customized fitness program.

A Wonderful Piece of Machinery

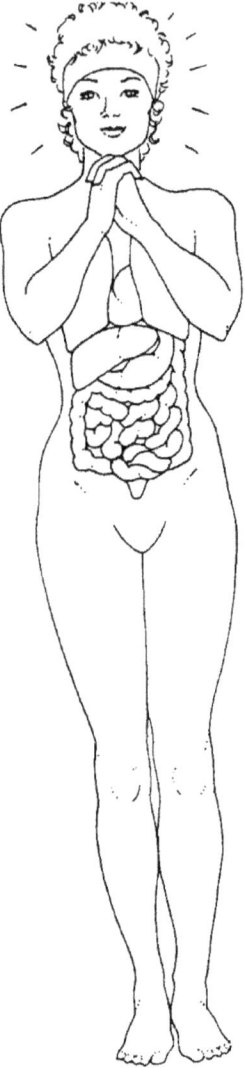

Your body is a remarkable, complex, and fascinating piece of machinery. It has mechanism upon mechanism for maintaining and repairing itself in times of breakdown. Consider as an example, a broken bone. A doctor sets the broken bone in place, immobilizes it, and your body does the rest. You don't have to take any medicine, except possibly for the prevention of infection. You just wait, and the body repairs the bone all by itself. When the mending is complete, the bone is actually stronger at the break than it was before you broke it. This phenomenon of repair is happening throughout the body on many different levels without our active participation. In some cases you can speed these processes or enhance their effectiveness. I hope that *Internal Fitness* will start you on an exciting road to a higher level of health.

Case Study - Ruby

Ruby was 37 years old when she discovered *Internal Fitness*. She was single, very attractive, and a talented musician. She had a very nice figure, except for being a little thick around the waist. Ruby had a magnificent head of prematurely gray hair, and a very alluring smile. Her smile was driven away almost weekly, however, by disabling migraine headaches. Constipation had been a problem for Ruby most of her adult life, and she had become quite dependent on laxatives. She took her Internal Fitness Evaluation and found that her first, second, and third areas of weakness were "a", "b", and "d", respectively. "a" and "b" were close together but "a" was in the lead, so Ruby started right away following the procedures from "a" and paying attention to the dietary suggestions. Ruby started her Internal Fitness Program during a migraine headache. Within 1 hour of the first workout her headache lightened, and within 24 hours it was totally gone. As far as I know, Ruby hasn't had another migraine. Within eight days of starting her fitness program, she was having daily bowel movements.

Ruby continued program "a" for 6 months. She was motivated to do so by the observation that after two months she had lost some weight, and was taking in her skirts at the waist. She also commented that a lot of the aches and pains to which she had become accustomed disappeared.

Case Study – Blake

Blake was somewhat of an entrepreneur on the island of Oahu. He worked for someone else, but it seemed as though all of the responsibility was his. He was the manager for several clothing stores and two book stores spread around the island. The stores were all owned by a Chinese-Hawaiian man who was very happy with the obvious fact that Blake was doing a job that should be handled by several people. Hours of every day Blake spent in heavy traffic getting from one store to another. Blake knew the job was too much for one person, but he was well paid, so he didn't complain. He knew getting a co-manager would cut into his salary.

Blake belonged to a fitness center that had branches in several locations on the island. About four days a week he was close enough to one of the branches to stop at lunchtime and workout on the Nautilus equipment. This kept Blake from getting totally stressed out.

He was now 42 years old, happily married with two children. He and his wife had always enjoyed being alone in the evenings in their bedroom after the kids had gone to sleep. They had maintained a very active love life for the duration of their marriage. There had been only brief intervals of inactivity when Blake was under so much stress that he would just pass out from exhaustion after dinner.

Over the past year, however, Blake had become increasingly unable to make love in the evenings. He and his wife were both disturbed by this turn of events, and were trying to manage as best they could, but neither knew exactly what to do about it.

In one of the book stores, he overheard a couple of the sales people talking about Internal Fitness. Blake wanted to jog or swim, but it was always nearly dark when he got through with work, and there certainly wasn't time during the day. The Internal Fitness Program looked like a good solution to Blake's lack of a fitness routine after work.

He scored "m" on his evaluation and started right away on the procedures. Blake noticed that he was feeling much less dragged out about one week into the program. Within 3 weeks, he was sort of feeling younger, more robust. After one month into the program, the bedroom started becoming a much more fun place again. Blake's wife was very happy with the Internal Fitness Program.

Case Study - Marilyn

Marilyn was 56 years old when she started her Internal Fitness program. She had always been very sedentary, had mostly worked as a secretary, had been married twice, and had one child. She had all of the symptoms of menopause, but they were mild and didn't interfere with her work schedule, so her doctor had decided against any treatment.

Marilyn started on her Internal Fitness program because it seemed to her that every time she looked into the mirror, she had a new wrinkle. She had handled aging fairly gracefully up to this point, but lately she had wondered if there wasn't some way to slow the process. Rejuvenation was what Marilyn was looking for.

Her evaluation score showed "k" as her primary area of weakness. She quickly got into the routine of doing the procedure daily, and modifying her diet as indicated for syndrome "k".

In a matter of days, she noticed that the late-in-the-day blahs had started to disappear. She also noticed that she was sleeping more soundly, and that the frequent adding and removing of blankets had lessened. Her body temperature seemed more stable. Over the course of the six months of internal body strengthening, Marilyn realized that she was no longer such a grouch at work. Her co-workers would comment on the change in her personality. She went on to strengthen the second and third areas of internal weakness, and was equally pleased with her results. Her Internal Fitness workout became part of Marilyn's life.

Case Study - Margie

Margie was a twenty nine year old artist. Her husband was ten years older and also an artist. They had a large studio in their house, and led, by most peoples' standards, a rather stress free life. They were very successful as artists. They received sizable fees for commission work, and put some hefty price tags on large pieces that they had worked on together.

Margie had always been pale and somewhat weak looking. One of her friends from Georgia always referred to her as "vaporish". Most of their friends just thought that artists are always like that because of working indoors and staying up late at night. She wasn't sick very often, and always said that she felt good. Marge did complain of getting tired easily.

Her husband teased her about being "allergic to exercise". He worried about her general health and endurance level. He got her interested in the Internal Fitness Program as something that she could do indoors at home. Her evaluation score showed "n" as her primary area of weakness. At first, Margie was alarmed when she saw that "n" was the Heart Meridian System. Her husband arrested her fears by explaining that the heart is basically a muscle. Like any other muscle, it can evidence different degrees of weakness or strength. The reason exercise enthusiasts do cardiovascular exercises is to strengthen the heart.

Margie started on the procedures and the dietary recommendations. At the end of two weeks, she looked like a different person. She had color in her cheeks, and seemed to have more light in her eyes. Margie often repeated the procedure, and modified her diet on a permanent basis. She continued to enjoy a strength that had not been there prior to the Internal Fitness program.

Mental Fitness As Well

In the Internal Fitness Program, you will be working primarily through the nervous system. Because of this, you can experience, as you progress, a greater sense of well being and a more relaxed feeling, while still having more energy and vitality. By fine tuning your nervous system, you are likely to experience greater mental fitness.

Purpose of the Book

The purpose of this book is to assist you in achieving your maximum potential on a physical and mental level. With *Internal Fitness*, you should be able to determine which of your internal organ systems is weak, and how to strengthen that system for optimum health. *Internal Fitness* is a manual with which you can, over a period of time, improve your internal health for a longer, healthier, more enjoyable life.

The information in this text, I have accumulated over a thirty-year period of studying nutrition, acupuncture, applied kinesiology, reflexology, meridian therapy, shiatsu, polarity, physical therapy, and chiropractic. One common message of these studies is that within you lies a wealth of untapped power that can be harnessed to achieve a higher state of being. In accordance with these sciences, the information in this book does not address sickness or disease. It is not to be interpreted as a substitute for proper medical care. All procedures in this book can be practiced concurrently with therapies and treatments prescribed by your physician.

Case Study – Kevin

Kevin was 27 years old when he was introduced to the Internal Fitness Program. He played sports everyday of his life, and had done so since his early teenage years. He was the youngest member of a very prestigious law firm, but his real love was playing racquet ball after work. For about a year prior to starting his Internal Fitness Program, he had been having a mysterious sharp pain in one shoulder. The pain was baffling many specialists, and for the past year he had been taking prescription pain medication, daily. Kevin was also having some stomach aches on a regular basis.

He started on the Internal Fitness Program, hoping that, somehow, it would lessen his shoulder pain. Kevin's scores were very low on his evaluation indicating that he was in pretty good shape, with the exception of "c" which was quite high. While on the fitness program, Kevin went to his orthopedic doctor for one of his routine exams regarding the shoulder. On hearing about the stomach complaints, the orthopedic specialist referred Kevin to an internist who diagnosed stomach ulcers as the problem. Kevin was given medication for the ulcers. He also continued with his Internal Fitness routine to strengthen his stomach. In a few weeks, he was off the ulcer medication, continued with his fitness program, and didn't have any more stomach difficulties.

His shoulder pain did not lessen and Kevin finally elected to have surgery. The internist who examined Kevin, had decided that the ulcer was caused by the amount of medication he had been taking to deal with the shoulder pain. After getting involved with his fitness program, Kevin was able to tolerate the same amount of pain medication without having his stomach bother him.

Ways To Use This Book

As evidenced in the case studies, Internal Fitness may be used to unravel many problems.

"Why can't I drop that last twenty pounds?"
"Why don't I have more energy even though I'm eating a healthier diet?"

For those of you who have successfully reached your diet and exercise goals, this book is the next logical step in personal physical achievement. As a fitness enthusiast with your muscle-to-fat ratio in a desirable place, you will want to attain new levels of excellence by getting your internal body as fit as your external body.

Find Your Weakest System

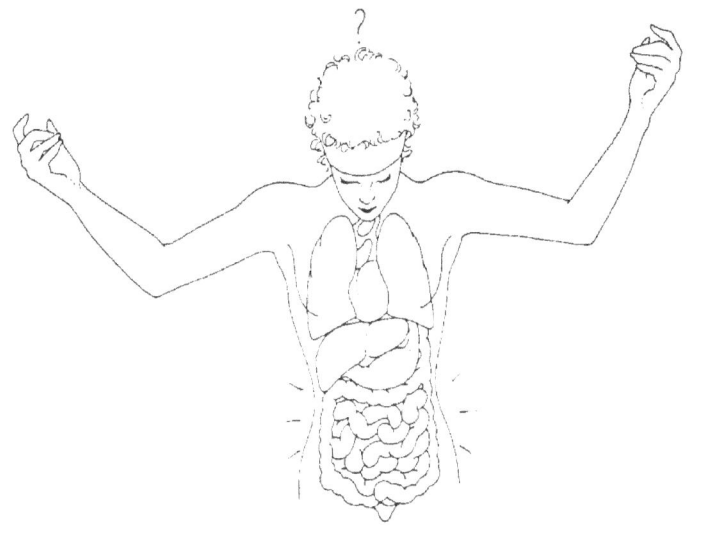

You can do this by finding, through your evaluation charts, the weakest system in your body and persistently working through the given procedures to elevate that system to its maximum potential. Or if you find, through the evaluation charts, that you do not have any particular weak areas, you can start on a total Internal Fitness Program, by systematically working through each of the body systems.

Case Study - Ron

Ron was a 42 year old massage therapist in Honolulu. I would occasionally get a massage from him after a busy day. He was always complaining of pain in his right shoulder. When he completed his Internal Fitness Evaluation, he was surprised and somewhat dismayed to find that a lot of his Meridian Systems showed up weak. Slightly weaker than the rest was his Gall Bladder Meridian System. After three days on the program the shoulder pain was gone, and Ron was increasing the number of massages he could do in a day. When he had finished the "b" section of his program, he became aware of the absence of the dull headaches which he had experienced every day for a month. He continued with the Internal Fitness Program, working his way through all of the organs that showed up weak on his evaluation. At one point, Ron told me that he was feeling better than he had in years, and that he believed he was "recreating himself".

Case Study - Estelle

Estelle was in her early 60's and in pretty good health, she thought. She had one problem that had bothered her for years, and was a real aggravation. She would get constipated quite often. She would take over the counter laxatives and immediately get diarrhea. She had been through numerous medical physical examinations and her tests always came back negative. Her Internal Fitness Evaluation indicated a weakness in area "d". Within two days of starting her new program, her bowel movements became more normal. As soon as she read through the program, Estelle realized that she had been eating all of the wrong foods. Some drastic changes were in order in the food department. In two weeks she was having normal daily bowel movements. She stopped the procedure at that point, but was always more reasonable with her diet. She was rarely bothered by irregular bowel movements, again.

Use Your Intuition

You have an intuitive sense of your own body that will guide you to a great extent in this process. Pay attention to this intuition. Realize when it may be time to discontinue a procedure prematurely, or rest for a while and continue later. Also, realize that this intuitive sense applies only to you. Never try to administer these procedures to someone else.

Case Study - Ellen

Ellen had been diagnosed by a naturopath and by a medical doctor as having Candidiasis (Systemic Candida Albicans). She had a myriad of mild physical symptoms and recurring vaginal yeast infections. She tried many treatments, most of which worked for a period of time, but the symptoms always eventually returned. A weak intestinal system was glaringly evident from Ellen's evaluation score sheet. It made sense to her that if the Candida had taken up housekeeping in her intestines so many times, that over the years her intestines would have been weakened.

Ellen was religious with her Internal Fitness Program. At the end of the first month, she could see great improvement in all of her complaints, and she had not had a vaginal yeast infection for the month. Since her problem had possibly been going on for years, I suggested that she take a break for a week or 10 days, follow the program for another month, take another break, and consider keeping this up for many months. She did this, and claimed that she felt generally better than she had for years. An increase in energy was the most noticeable result of her program.

Case Study – Dale

Dale was a 37 year old environmental engineer from California. He had always been a good athlete. He enjoyed running as his primary form of exercise because it was most convenient to his lifestyle. Most of his college buddies had families, now, and, in his opinion, had gotten out of shape. They had, one by one, dropped out of competitive sports, so he was left to get involved in individual sports.

It was easy to see why Dale was still single. He was either working or running. Five or ten miles a day was average for Dale. When you add that amount of time to a 40 hour work week, there are few hours left for romance. If he ever slowed down long enough for single women to get a look at him, however, the interest in women's track might have taken a sudden leap forward.

Dale was tall and handsome, with a ruddy complexion and a remarkable physique. He really didn't look over twenty-five except for some gray in his thick, dark hair. Dale never had any physical complaints and was never sick. He was interested in the Internal Fitness Program because he felt as though he had reached a plateau in his conditioning. He wanted to move on to greater heights of physical achievement.

Dale's evaluation showed him weak in area "f". He thought this was strange since he never had back pain and had always heard about kidney problems causing back pain. Dale had been planning to just start with section "a", and work his way through the book, stimulating all of the organ areas to increase his overall fitness potential. I convinced him to go through the evaluation, and he was very pleased that he had. Stimulating his kidneys made a big difference in his endurance level as a runner, almost immediately. He realized, in the process of strengthening his kidneys, that he had not been drinking enough water for the amount of exercise he was doing.

Folk Medicine

Our great grandparents had an extensive knowledge of home remedies and health practices that were passed down to them from their parents. These potions and tonics served them well in the absence of modern medicine. Mostly, they realized that serious illness might result in death. With this in mind, they tried very hard not to get sick. Your grandparents were conditioned to practice certain health maintenance procedures daily to keep from becoming ill.

Wonder Drugs

Since the advent of sulfa drugs in the 1940's, conditioning about health has changed greatly. People have been allowed to take much less responsibility for their own health. Sulfa drugs meant that if you became very ill, you would take medicine and be returned to good health in short order. Many lives were saved, but our concept of health maintenance was changed as well. Maintaining good health through daily health practices gave way to ignoring health until a crisis arose. *Internal Fitness* may empower you with the option of taking more responsibility for your own health.

Case Study – Penny

Penny was 39 years old and in very good physical condition. As a jogger, she was faithful to her routine of running two miles every other day. Occasionally she would get what she considered normal aches and pains as she pressed her muscles on for more. Usually this wasn't too bothersome as long as she stretched before and after exercise.

For two years, she had noticed the same aching sensation in her right hip after running. It wasn't very painful, just a mild ache. Her hip had been examined by a specialist, but the exam findings reported a normal hip. The aching sensation never got worse or better, it was just there. Every six months, or so, her doctor would give her a check up, but nothing ever showed up on the tests.

Penny was interested in *Internal Fitness* because she wanted to be sure that she was working as hard on the inside of her body as the outside. She didn't really think about her hip when she started her internal strengthening. She assumed that her hip problem was a musculoskeletal problem. Her score sheet wasn't very dramatic on evaluation, but it did point out that she needed strengthening in area "g".

By the time she had completed the three weeks of procedure, Penny thought that the aching in her hip was less after her runs. She didn't associate it with the Internal Fitness Program right away, but it continued to get better even after she finished the procedure, and was only doing her diet modification. By the end of the two month period, the hip aching was virtually gone. Penny was ecstatic, and once again became a happy runner.

Invest In Health

There is no better investment than your health. A little time and a little money invested on a daily basis toward improving your health picture will pay dividends that you will enjoy as long you live. You will experience more quality to your days and you will have more days to enjoy quality living.

Case Study – Grant

Grant was 20 years old. His parents introduced him to Internal Fitness because he was always tired and just moped around the house. They were hoping that this would give him some extra energy, or at least give him a new interest.

Grant wasn't too excited at first, but after reading about the program, he thought that he might be able to improve his bad skin. He had started having facial acne in his mid-teens, and it had not gotten much better as he aged. All the acne goops from the drug store hadn't helped very much.

His evaluation showed that he might have a weakness in his pancreas. Grant had never heard of his pancreas, and wasn't too interested in getting familiar with it, but started the program, anyway. Within three days he was pretty sure that he had more energy. Within ten days his skin was noticeably better. After 2 weeks, Grant was happy to be finished with the procedure part of the program. At this time he also quit the nutritional segment because he missed his comfort foods.

His skin stayed clear for a couple of weeks, and then he started to break out again. This made Grant pretty mad. His parents had to review a subject with him that they had been over many times. They reminded him that sometimes you have to stick to things awhile in order to get results. They also pointed out to their son that as soon as his skin started clearing up he started eating more junk. Over the course of the next six weeks, Grant learned a little more about self discipline. He went through the procedure three times and found that his skin stabilized with a very healthy looking complexion. It was never clear to his parents whether it was the Internal Fitness Program that raised his energy level, or the skin improvement that got him out of the house, but the final outcome was pleasant for everyone involved.

Case Study – Harold

Harold was 63, and didn't really have too many complaints. He had been pretty sedentary all of his life, having always worked desk jobs. He had annual check-ups from his doctor, and had never had any alarming results. The Internal Fitness Program appealed to Harold simply because he wasn't an exerciser, and felt guilty about never doing much to stay in shape.

When his fitness evaluation was complete, Harold was surprised to have scored an "i" as his area of major weakness. He had expected his heart to show up weak, only because he was 63 years old. He scheduled his annual physical early, so that he could get his medical doctor to check on his prostate. The doctor found that in fact, Harold had a slightly enlarged prostate gland, but "nothing abnormal for his age". His doctor assured him that it was nothing to be concerned about. Harold never liked it when he was told that problems were "normal for his age". To Harold it sounded too much like "over the hill". Since Harold wasn't really having complaints, he didn't know what to look for in the way of results. But he did like the idea of strengthening an area that he thought was a problem.

As time went on, Harold found that he enjoyed the program. He repeated it many times. Harold was quite sure that it improved his general sense of well-being.

Case Study – Mildred

Mildred was a "special ed" teacher in a public school. She was married and had two pre-teenage girls. Anyone who has been in a special education public school classroom, or has pre-teenage girls, can tell you that Mildred's life was not easy. She was now 36 years old, and had been a smoker since her late teenage years. She knew that smoking was bad for her health, and contributed to many of her health problems. Mildred felt that smoking allowed her to deal with the stress that seemed to dominate her life. She had tried to quit a couple of times, but it always made her want to eat more, and consequently gain weight. She was an active tennis and golf player, so the idea of gaining weight was no more appealing than smoking.

Every winter Mildred had one respiratory difficulty after another. As winter progressed, so did her sinus infections, colds, flu, bronchitis, and finally pneumonia. It was the pneumonia that made her realize that she had to do something.

System "j" was a standout on her evaluation score. Mildred found it convenient to perform the procedure just before going to bed. The slight dietary changes she could handle without difficulty during her busy day.

Mildred adopted her internal fitness program as a new part of her life. It was something positive that she did for herself every day, among all the negative events that she seemed to be up against in her daily schedule. It was something that she could incorporate without having to alter her lifestyle, which was a nice change from the other health improving plans she had embarked upon in the past. Mildred continued to chauffeur her teenagers, work more than full time, and play tennis and golf. She continued her hectic life, but with greater vitality and fewer sick days.

Your Internal Body Strength

Most people go through their daily routine with subtle but annoying physical complaints that don't actually reflect illness, but indicate that things could be better. A trip to the doctor may reveal the presence of an illness resulting in treatment prescribed and the problem corrected. But many times, particularly with the more non-specific complaints, the doctor's exam reports come back negative, indicating that nothing is wrong. This is very good news. This means that you have no sickness or disease, as reported by the laboratory results and physical exam.

But what about those annoying little complaints that caused you to seek medical evaluation in the first place? My experience has led me to believe that many of these can be tracked to a weakness in one of the body's internal systems. Just as a muscle gets tired and weak and doesn't perform well, so do internal organs and glands. Common complaints that can indicate weakness of internal systems include:

-general or specific mild aches and pains
-headaches
-fluctuating energy levels
-thermal discomfort
-body odors
-poor skin color or texture
-fatigue, sleeplessness, lethargy

Now, in the Internal Fitness Program, you have a system for determining which areas of your body are weak, and how you can, over a period of time, strengthen these areas.

The Viscerosomatic Reflex

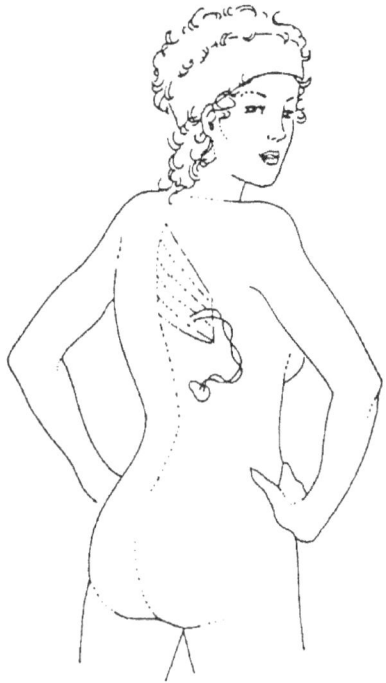

In clinical studies, I have found that there is often a weakness in some organ system of the body. This weakness blocks the continuation of physical progress. Once the internal system in question has been strengthened, the expected results can be realized. This process takes place through the communicating mechanisms of the nervous system. You have, in your body, an action called a viscerosomatic reflex, whereby a weak organ causes a weakness to take place in a corresponding muscle. This event takes place in a highly organized fashion, each organ having a specific muscle group that it affects.

For example, a weakness in your gall bladder will cause a corresponding weakness in the right rhomboid muscle which connects your shoulder blade to the spinal column. Consequently, if you have a weakness in the gall bladder, you may experience problems with that right shoulder and arm. You may not be able to get as much work out of the arm, either on an everyday activity level or from a muscle development standpoint. Strengthening the internal organ removes the weak viscerosomatic reflex, eliminating the muscle problem of the shoulder.

Weakness Not Illness

Keep in mind that I have not mentioned any gall bladder symptoms. This viscerosomatic reflex happens even in the absence of gall bladder distress or illness. I am only addressing a condition of weakness or laziness in the organ. Strengthening your internal organ system will allow you to proceed farther with your health goals. This is true whether your interest is body building or feeling better all of the time.

Work For Results

In the next few chapters, you will evaluate your weak areas, decide on procedures for strengthening those areas, and follow through with those procedures. You should then wait a few weeks before going through the evaluation procedure again. You may wish to repeat the fitness routine two or three times before moving on to the next area of weakness. Keep in mind that due to lifestyle, illness, and stress, you may develop other weakness that would change your results on a subsequent evaluation.

Diet, Exercise and Weight Loss

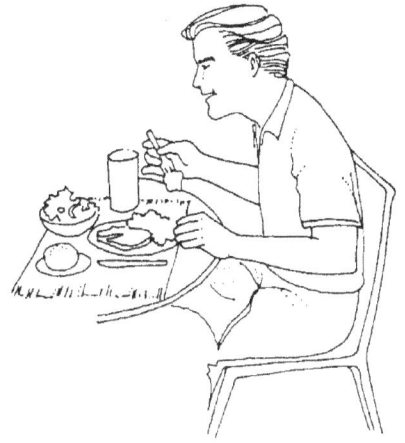

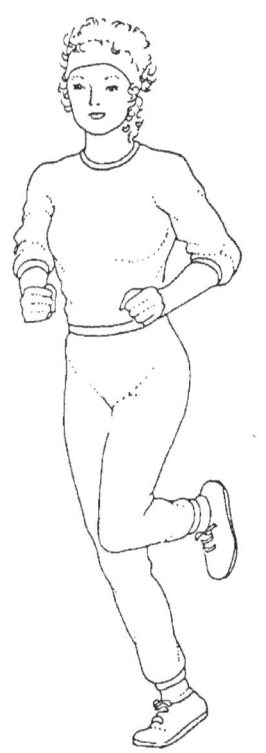

There are hundreds of diet books on the market. They sell because people are hoping for a straight forward approach to weight loss. Unfortunately, no one lost weight reading a book.

The perfect diet/weight loss book should be two paragraphs in length. In spite of the plethora of diet books, our national obesity problem continues to increase. Diet books have served to divert the readers' attention from what they really need to do.

So, here is my two paragraph weight loss book. If you do this, you will assume your normal body weight and stay there. That should be your key goal, not just losing weight, but keeping it off.

Paragraph 1.
Diet: Eat fresh fruits and vegetables (mostly vegetables), lean meat, nuts, seeds and fish. Eat as many vegetables as you want; eat moderate amounts of the other foods. Stay away from white foods (bread, pasta, rice, potatoes, sugar). Eliminate sodas, fried food and anything that contains sugar. Do not drink liquids with meals.
Paragraph 2.
Exercise: Commit to one hour of vigorous, age-appropriate exercise every day. Be creative. Make it fun. Get a buddy or partner involved. Don't use weather as an excuse to skip a day.

If you can discipline yourself to follow this two-paragraph protocol, you can achieve your weight loss goals. The Internal Fitness program may make this process easier and faster. By strengthening your internal organs your body is able to more easily go through the processes necessary for weight loss.

Body Strengthening

It is important in reading that you understand that this book will not diagnose illness or disease of any kind. The procedures detailed on the following pages are for body strengthening only, and are not to be interpreted as a substitute for diagnosis or treatment by a qualified physician, should illness be suspected.

Pay Attention To Your Body

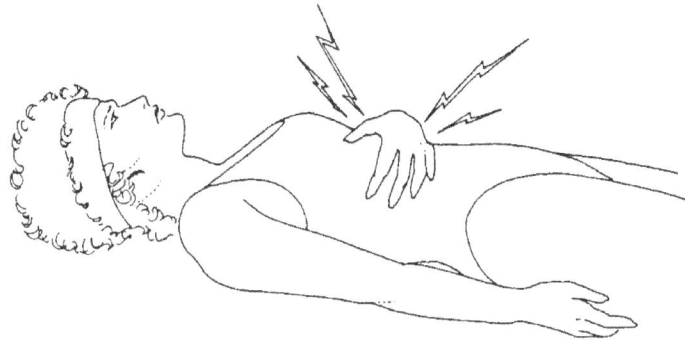

All of the body-strengthening procedures in this book are totally painless. Should you experience any pain while performing these procedures, you may have a physical disorder or condition that needs the attention of a physician. In that case, seek the consultation of a qualified physician, and discontinue the procedure, immediately, until you have resolved the source of your pain. If during the course of performing a procedure in this book, you notice that your complaints get worse, you should discontinue that procedure at once, and seek professional care. You may be dealing with illness rather than internal organ weakness.

Every Body Is Different

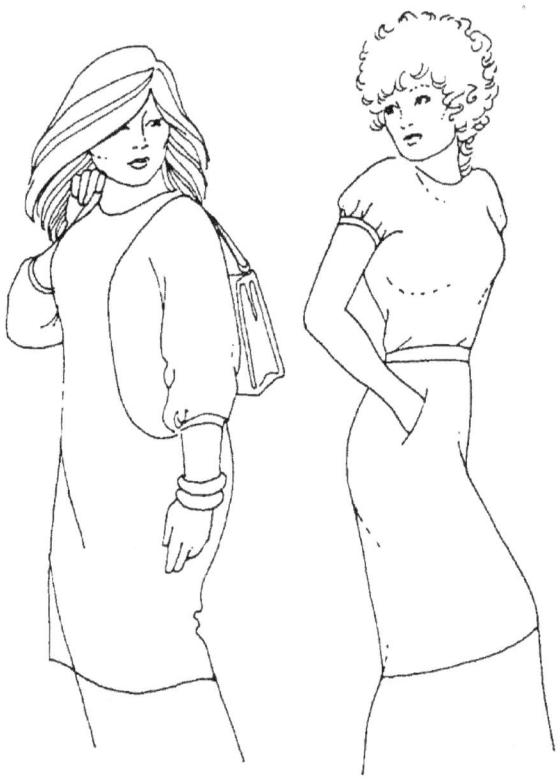

When working with the human body, there are various guidelines to direct us, but you ultimately have to realize that responses vary, and that there are no absolutes. I hope that you will respond quickly and directly to your internal body strengthening regime. Some, however, will get results slowly, and some not at all. Such is the nature of humans. This book is certainly not a guarantee of elevated internal health, but rather the next step in your efforts to maintain fitness and improve your general quality of life.

Getting Started

When involved in a health conversation, I am frequently asked, "Where do I start?" So often, people assume a daily routine that includes many bad habits. Changing lifestyle to opt for more emphasis on health can look like an impossible task. My suggestion is to make a list of habits that you consider bad from a health standpoint.

Read over this list, and select one which you feel can be eliminated for good. Realize that getting rid of just one habit will improve your health, and that an improvement in your health is invaluable. Work on your attitude about eliminating this habit. Consider that it is a totally positive action, not a deprivation. If you do this, you will form a solid commitment to rid your life of this one health-eroding habit. Be sure, in doing this, to select a habit that you can realistically break. Don't choose the most difficult habit on your list for elimination. Choose one that, given your life style at this particular time, you can eliminate without great sacrifice. Otherwise, you could be setting yourself up for failure. Any bad habit broken is an improvement in your health, so be realistic in your task.

Bad Habits

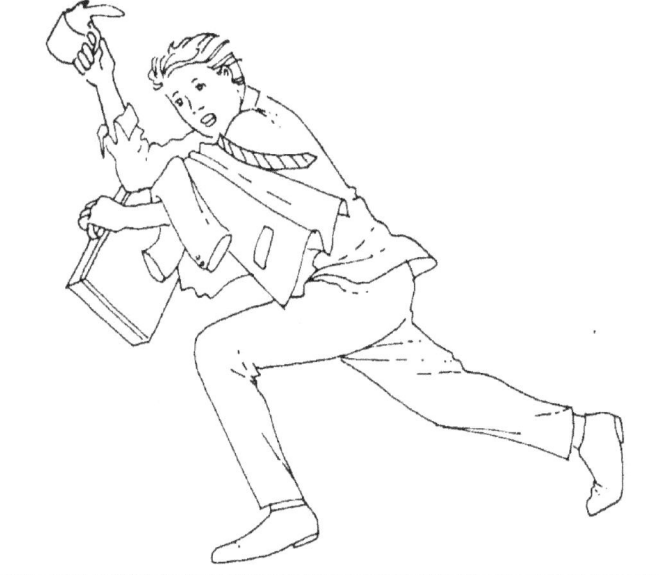

Common single bad habits that are good candidates for elimination include:

Midnight Snack

Eating late into the night overloads the digestive system when your metabolism is at its slowest. This leaves many unburned calories.

Skipping Breakfast

Not eating breakfast creates an imbalance in blood sugar levels. This makes you hungry later in the day. It also creates dips and peaks in your energy level throughout the day.

Drinking With Meals

Drinking large amounts of liquid with meals dilutes hydrochloric acid and other biochemicals for digestion of food. This makes your digestive system less efficient. Carbonated drinks interfere with the process of digestion by neutralizing stomach acidity. This includes soft drinks, carbonated mineral water, and beer.

Cigarette Smoking

I realize that this is easier said than done for the habitual smoker. Smoking is a real drag on the whole body. By introducing toxic matter, smoking slows down many body functions.

Pick Up A Good Habit

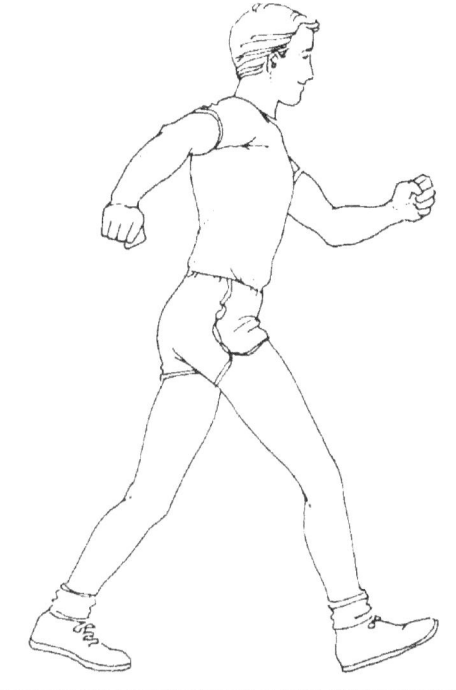

While you are eliminating your bad habit, why not add one good habit to your daily routine. If you do, you have just improved your health even further. Common single good habits that can be easily added to daily activities include:

Drinking More Water During The Day

Six to eight glasses of water per day (not soft drinks) clean the kidneys, assist with elimination of waste, and maintain proper chemical balance in the body.

Getting Some Exercise Every Day

Park the car and walk on some of your errands. Walking with a destination is one of the best forms of exercise.

Have Your Drinking Water Tested

If it's not good quality, have a water purification system installed in your home, or get a portable model if you live in an apartment.

Eliminate Candy Bars And Cookies

Don't buy them. If you don't have them around, you can't eat them. Eat fresh or dried fruit for snacks.

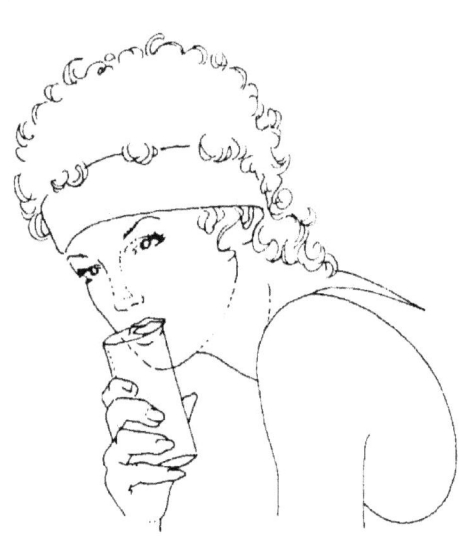

27

The Evaluation
The Evaluation Score Sheet.

System   Score

a									
b									
c									
d									
e									
f									
g									
h									
i									
j									
k									
m									
n									

_____ 1st   _____ 2nd   _____ 3rd System

Create a form identical or similar to the one on the previous page. In the following chapters, you will need to record the number of times that you scored the letters "a" through "n". Every time you score a letter, put a check mark beside the letter. This is a simple process, but it can get confusing if you don't use the Evaluation Score Sheet. Dating the sheet will allow you to compare progress made between evaluations.

The letter of the alphabet on your Evaluation Score Sheet that received the most check marks is your area of greatest weakness. Write this letter on your Evaluation Score Sheet where it says "1st SYSTEM" for easy future reference. Also notice letters that may have received nearly as many check marks as your first letter. Mark these on your Evaluation Score Sheet as second or third weaknesses.

The Complaint Chart

Read the following list of complaints. As you read, ask yourself, "Have I experienced this complaint many times over the past six months?" If the answer is "yes", then put a check mark on your evaluation sheet by the letter or letters of the alphabet that corresponds to the letter or letters at the end of the complaint.

Example:
 right shoulder tension = b,d
You would put a check mark by both "b" and "d" on your evaluation sheet if this is a complaint that you have experienced many times in the past six months.

Read each of the following complaints. Be careful not to skip any. This would seriously affect your score. Mark the applicable letters on your evaluation sheet.

1. sinus congestion and scratchy throat = j
2. discomfort in right upper abdomen = b
3. right shoulder tightness = b,d
4. tightness on the top of the left shoulder = c
5. discomfort in the stomach = c
6. discomfort just under the rib cage = h,e
7. discomfort to the right of the sternum (breast bone) = h

8. discomfort in the center of the forehead = g
9. discomfort in the lower right side of the abdomen = g
10. tightness in the center of the right buttock = g
11. discomfort around the navel = e
12. back discomfort just above the waistline = e,f
13. discomfort on the inside of the elbows toward the fingers = e
14. swelling of one ankle = f
15. dry or cracked lips = f
16. ringing in the ears = d
17. uncomfortable metatarsals = d
18. discomfort across the lower part of the abdomen = a
19. tightness in the lower part of both hips = a
20. discomfort behind both ears = i
21. discomfort on the inside of both ankles = i
22. discomfort in the pubic area = i,k
23. tightness in both thighs = i,k
24. discomfort across the middle of the back = m
25. arthritic feeling in hands = m
26. tighness between the shoulder blades just to the right of the spinal column = h
27. chronic cough or sneeze = j
28. post nasal drip = j
29. sinus headaches = j
30. headache that wraps around the back of the head from the bottom of the skull to the ears = h
31. migraine headache = d
32. headache in back of the head at the top = a
33. headache on waking that goes away after morning urination = f
34. chronic neck stiffness = a, c
35. tightening in shoulders = b
36. cold hands and feet = m
37. loss of sleep = m
38. nervousness = m
39. chronic fatigue = n
40. belching or gas = d, e, b
41. nausea = c
42. hemorrhoids = g
43. rapid or slow heart beat = n
44. high blood pressure = n

45. discomfort in center of chest = n
46. swelling of both ankles = n
47. varicose veins = g
48. frequent skin eruptions = a
49. dryness of skin = m
50. short of breath = n
51. frequent urination = f
52. constipation = a,d

For Men Only
53. loss of libido = m
54. pain during intercourse or ejaculation = i

For Women Only
55. sore, tender breasts = k
56. painful periods = k
57. menstrual cramps = k

The Reflex Scan

Read each numbered item in the Reflex Scan. Perform each reflex testing procedure as you read, and if you have a tender reflex, mark the indicated letter on your Evaluation Score Sheet. You may want to refer to the diagrams at the end of this section for assistance in locating the reflexes. Each item on the Reflex Scan describes the location of a point or combination of points on your body. For the most part, you will be pressing on these points to check for tenderness. Press several times to give the reflex a good test. Sometimes the tenderness will show up as you are taking your finger off the point. If tenderness is present, it will be quite evident. If you are uncertain, then you probably do not have an active reflex at that point.

1. Locate a reflex point one inch from the body center line and one and one half inches down from the bottom of the collarbone (clavicle). This reflex is positive if the right side is noticeably more tender than the left = g

2. Lightly squeeze, with your fingers, the outermost part of the collarbone (clavicle). Now lightly squeeze the innermost part of the collarbone. If there is a noticeable difference in tenderness between the outer and inner pair of points (the outer pair aren't tender, but the two inside reflexes are very sensitive or vice versa) = a

3. Let your arm fall limp to your side. Run your index finger up the arm to the top, front, of the arm bone. Roll your finger around on the front of the shoulder. Press at the center of this point. Compare right and left. If the right side is noticeably more tender = d

4. Approximate the middle of the collarbone on both sides of the body. Press one inch below each collarbone, then two inches below each collarbone, then three inches below each collarbone. There are six points in all, and they are between the ribs. If two or more of the points are tender = j

5. On a vertical line halfway between the midline and the right side of the body, find the bottom of the rib cage. Come straight up two inches and press on that rib. If tender = b

6. Reflex points are located on both sides of the body one inch up from the naval and four inches to either side. Press with five or six pounds of pressure so that the skin over the abdomen is depressed a couple of inches. If either side is tender = f

7. Reflex points are one inch above and one inch below the naval. Either one tender = e

8. (FEMALE ONLY) From the top of the pelvic bone on one side to the top of the pubic bone on the same side imagine a line. Along this line, there two long reflexes. If any of the four (two each side) are tender = k

9. Spread the fingers of your hands so that the thumb and forefinger form a "V". Squeeze the fleshy area at the bottom of this "V". Compare the tenderness of these areas.

Right hand more tender = b
Left hand more tender = c

10. On the palm face of the hand, press into the base of the thumb where it is actually part of the body of the hand (thenar pad). Compare right and left hands.

Right hand more tender = h
Left hand more tender = n

11. Locate large area reflex points on the top of both feet near the toes. Both feet must be tender = j

12. Reflex points are on the back of the feet just above the heel (squeeze the Achilles tendon). If both right and left points are tender = i, k

13. Locate a reflex point on the bottom of the right foot 2 to 2 ½ inches from (little) toes. If tender = g

14. Locate a reflex point on right foot bottom 2 to 2 ½ inches from middle toes. If tender = h

15. From the center of the arch on the bottom of the foot, find a point one inch toward the toes and one inch from the inside edge of the foot. If this point is tender, either foot = f

16. Find a point 3 inches to the left of the body centerline and 2 inches below the rib cage. If this point if tender = c

17. Find a point on the left bottom rib, midway between the body centerline and the side of the body. If tender = h

18. Find a point under the last rib on the right, midway between the body centerline and the side of the body. If tender = h

19. (FOR MEN ONLY) Find a point midway between the rectum and the scrotum. If tender =i

20. Immediately under the earlobes, press into the neck with your index fingers opposing each other. Tender reflex either side = j

21. On the bottom of both feet, press 2-2 1/2 inches from the base of the big toe. If tender on both feet = c

22. On the bottom of both feet, press the area between the center of the arch and the heel. If tender either foot = e

When you have finished with the Complaints Chart and the Reflex Scan, and recorded your results on the Evaluation Score Sheet, your evaluation is complete. The letter of the alphabet on your Evaluation Score Sheet that received the most check marks is your area of greatest weakness. Write this letter on your Evaluation Score Sheet where it says "1st SYSTEM" for easy future reference. Also notice letters that may have received nearly as many check marks as your first letter. Mark these on your Evaluation Score Sheet as second or third weaknesses.

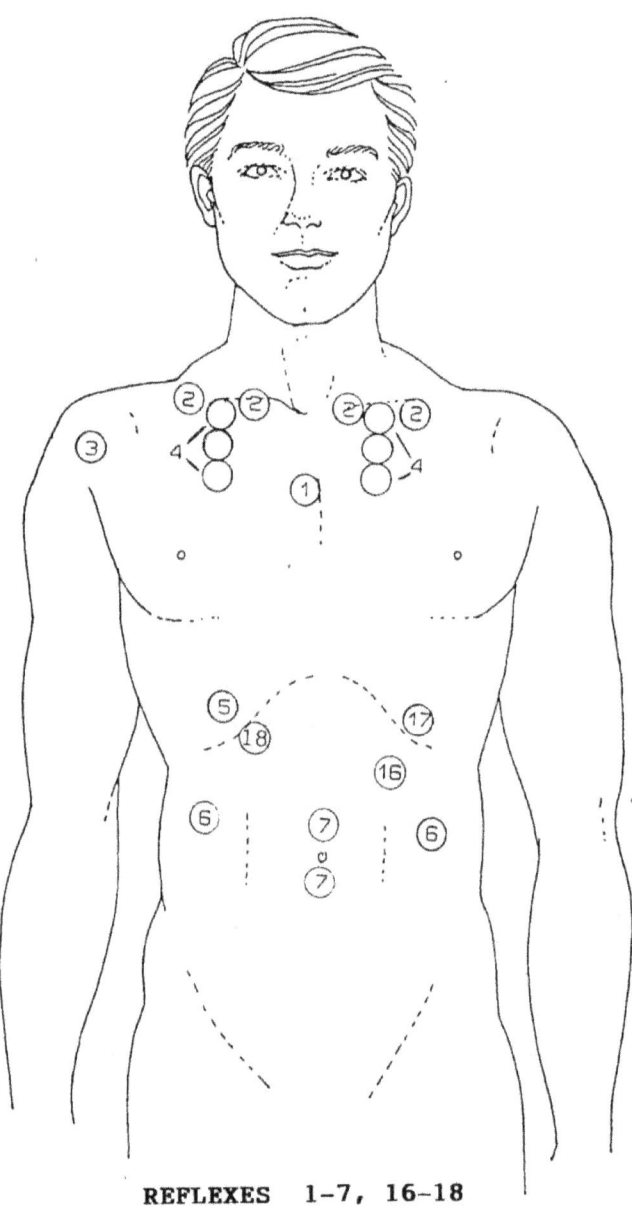

REFLEXES 1–7, 16–18

Use the above diagram to locate reflexes 1 through 7 and 16 through 18.

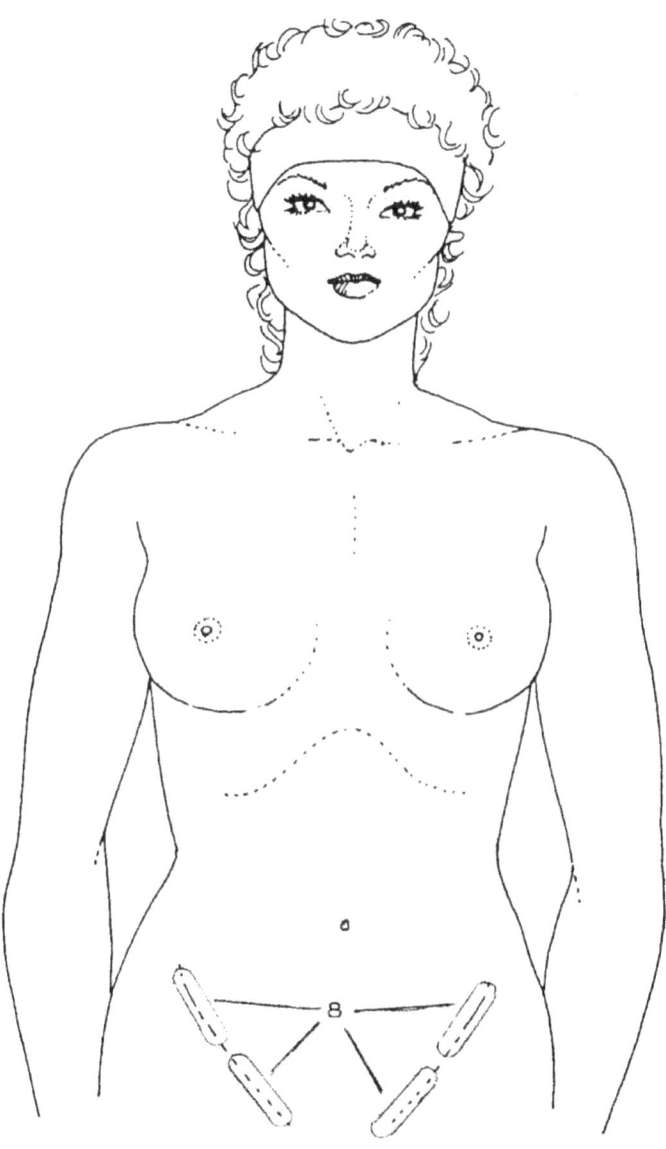

REFLEX 8

Use the above diagram to locate reflex 8.

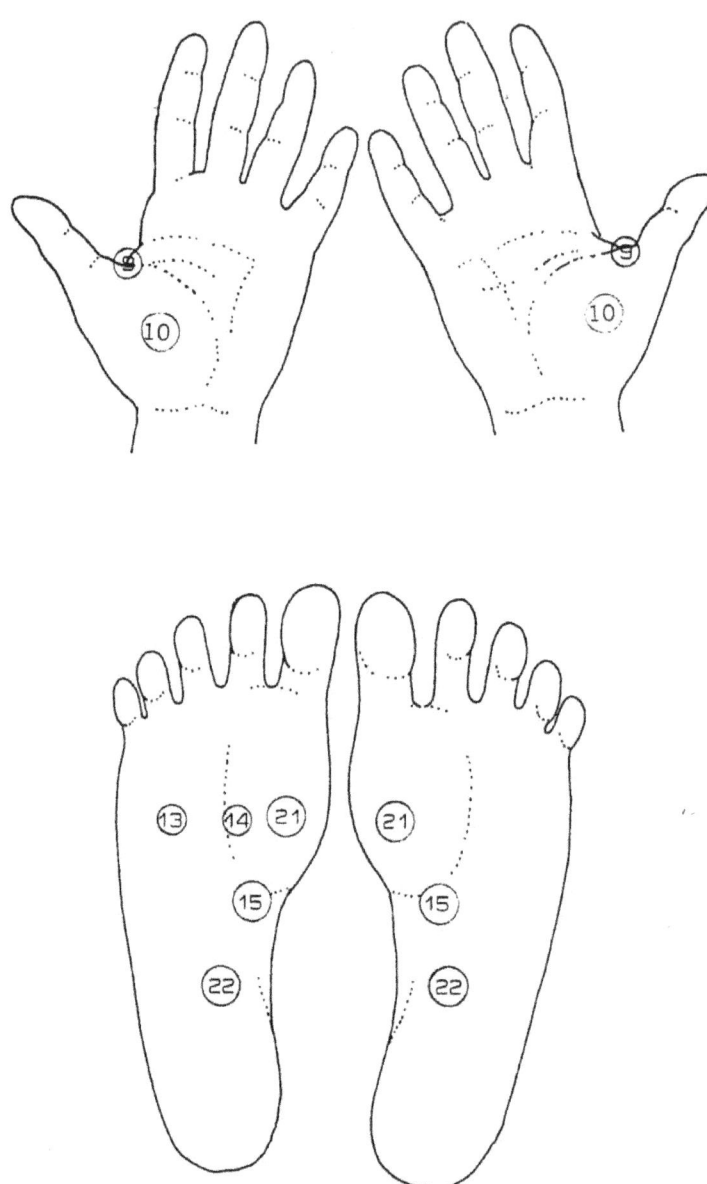

REFLEXES 9, 10, 13–15, 21, 22

Use the above chart to locate reflexes 9, 10, 13, 14, 15, 21 and 22.

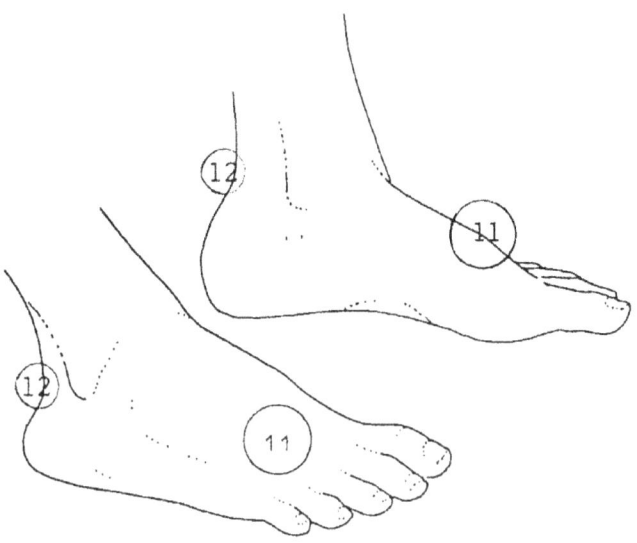

Use the above diagram to locate reflexes 11 and 12.

Internal Health Systems

This section lists the Internal Systems by alphabetical letters. Find the area that corresponds to the letter that you wrote on your Evaluation Score Sheet as your primary weakness. You will find here the following information:

A. The location of the organ or gland that is of major importance in this internal meridian system in your body.

B. The function of the organ or gland that is of major importance in this system.

C. The general effect of a weakness in that system. There are many effects of such a weakness. I have tried to describe some of the major ones.

D. The procedure for strengthening your weak body system.

Get Comfortable

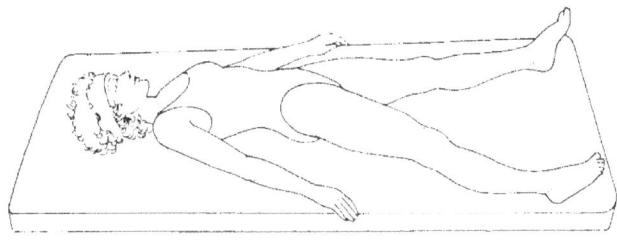

The procedure in this section must be performed in the order stated. You should be lying down in a comfortable room on a comfortable, but firm, surface. Do not lie down on a cold, hard floor or a sagging bed. You should start your procedure by relaxing in this position for a few minutes. Feel the surface you are on pressing into your back. This few minutes of relaxation allows areas of stagnant energy in your body to open up. Once you start your procedure, take your time. Make sure that you are correctly locating all of the points. This is important because you will be repeating the procedure in your fitness program, just as you would walk, jog, swim, or row repeatedly.

Throughout the procedure sections, reference is made to the amount of pressure applied to reflex points. The amount of pressure suggested varies from 1 to 6 pounds. To help you estimate this pressure, consider this: if you were pressing on a ripe banana with your thumb, 1 pound of pressure would hardly dent the banana. Three pounds of pressure would indent, but not break the skin. Six pounds of pressure would break the skin of the banana.

Allow Time For Nature To Work

After you have completed the designated procedure and dietary considerations, stop and take time to consider your results. If you feel worse than when you started, you should consult a physician about your condition. You may be dealing with illness rather than weakness. If you don't feel considerably different than when you

41

started, you should start this program again, and see if a second or third workout with the same procedures produces results.

If, on the other hand, your results have been dramatic, you should give yourself a rest of a few days, and then start on procedures for your second area of weakness as indicated on your evaluation sheet.

At least every three months, you should go through the entire evaluation procedure from the start so that you have a graphic idea of your progress. This will also make you aware of any new areas of weakness that may need strengthening.

The Systems

Colon Meridian System (a)

A. Your colon occupies the lower part of your abdomen, and runs from side to side.

B. The final stage of food digestion takes place here. The colon is responsible for the transfer of solid waste material from food digestion by peristalsis.

C. If the colon is not functioning, properly, waste toxins may be reabsorbed into the blood stream or food material released from the body before all nutrients are extracted from it.

D. PROCEDURE.

Lie down on your back on the floor or a firm bed. With your finger, trace an ellipse (flattened circle) between your naval, pubic bone, and sides. Using both hands, massage along this line in a clockwise direction with medium pressure. See diagram, next page. You may find some very tender spots as you traverse the abdomen. These areas will become less tender as the procedure progresses. Should the tender spots become more tender as you proceed from day to day, discontinue the procedure, and consult a physician. This procedure should be performed once a day for three minutes duration for a two week period. Discontinue for one week, and then proceed for two more weeks. Continue this pattern until complaints and reflexes subside.

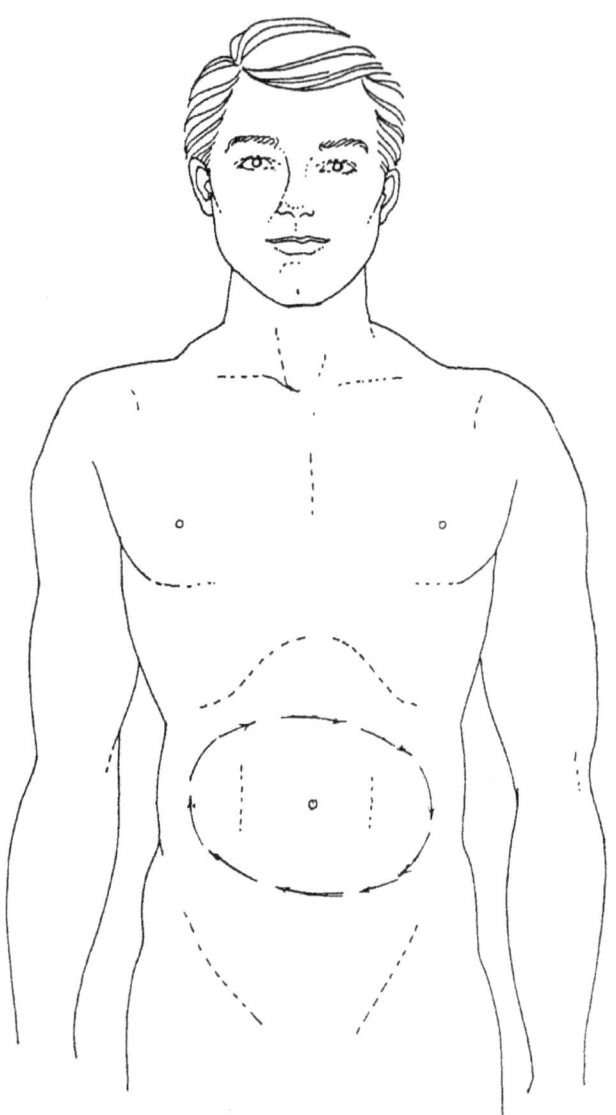

COLON MERIDIAN SYSTEM

If chronic diarrhea is a problem, reverse the direction of massage. That is, move the fingers in a counterclockwise direction along the same ellipse. Otherwise follow all of the same procedures. If discomfort occurs, during or after this process, discontinue the procedure.

Foods To Avoid - fried meats, overcooked foods
Foods To Include - Eat more fiber such as raw fruits and vegetables, wheat bran, and whole grains. Exercise is important in proper colon function. If you are not getting regular exercise, do so. Walking is especially beneficial.

Gall Bladder Meridian System (b)

A. The gall bladder is located just underneath the right rib cage. It is just forward of the liver.

B. The gall bladder stores bile which is produced by the liver. When you eat fats, the gall bladder releases bile into the duodenum to help breakdown the fats, thus aiding digestion.

C. If the gall bladder is sluggish, digestion will be slowed down and sometimes left incomplete. If you have a weak gall bladder you are likely to gain weight easily, particularly at the waist line, without overeating. Likewise, you may find it difficult to lose weight even when food intake is restricted. Many discomforts associated with indigestion accompany a weak gall bladder, including frequent headaches.

D. PROCEDURE

Since the gall bladder is activated by food intake, it is effective to strengthen with nutrition. Take one tablespoon of cold pressed, extra virgin olive oil first thing in the morning on an empty stomach. Wait 20 minutes before eating or drinking. If the taste is unpleasant, brush your teeth and tongue afterwards. Do this every morning for 5 days, if you can tolerate the taste. If not, discontinue and proceed with manually stimulating the gall bladder.

Cup the right hand over the right rib cage so that the fingers curl under the last rib and pressing into the abdomen and slightly up. Leave the fingers pressing lightly into the abdomen and breathe deeply. This may be fairly uncomfortable. As you breathe deeply leave the fingers in place, so that the stomach presses into them. Keep the fingers there for 5 deep breaths. Do this twice a day for 2 weeks. If discomfort occurs, during or after this process, discontinue the procedure.

Foods To Avoid - Pork, fried foods, lard or shortening, alcohol, coffee
Foods To Include - Safflower oil for cooking and salad dressings, lean beef, fish, bread, vegetables, pears, beets.

Stomach Meridian System (c)

A. The stomach is located just below your rib cage on the left side of the abdomen.

B. The stomach is the first major area of digestion for the food you eat. Rich in hydrochloric acid (HCL), it prepares your ingested meal for its passage through the small and large intestine.

C. A malfunctioning stomach usually results in a great deal of discomfort. Belching, gas, and other signs of indigestion accompany a distressed stomach. The whole process of digestion is literally off to a bad start with the stomach system.

D. PROCEDURE

Locate the reflex points on the bottom of the feet shown on the figure on the following page. These areas will probably be tender to the exertion of medium thumb pressure (about 5 lbs.). Massage one point and then the other for about 3 minutes each using a rotary motion of your thumb and medium pressure (3 to 5 lbs.). During this procedure, breathe slowly and deeply to maximize oxygen intake. Now open your left hand so that the fingers are spread apart. Relax the hand and grab the reflex point, shown on the figure, with your thumb and index finger. This point is about 3/4 inches from the outside intersection the thumb and forefinger. Squeeze this reflex point with medium pressure (3 to 5 lbs.). Squeeze with a rotary motion for 3 minutes. The point will be very tender.

Do this procedure (both feet and hand) every day for one month. If discomfort occurs, during or after this process, discontinue the procedure.

Foods To Avoid - tobacco, alcohol, coffee, tea, chocolate, salt, white and black pepper, mustard, vinegar, chili, white sugar, soft drinks, and carbonated waters

Foods To Include - cabbage, potatoes, yogurt

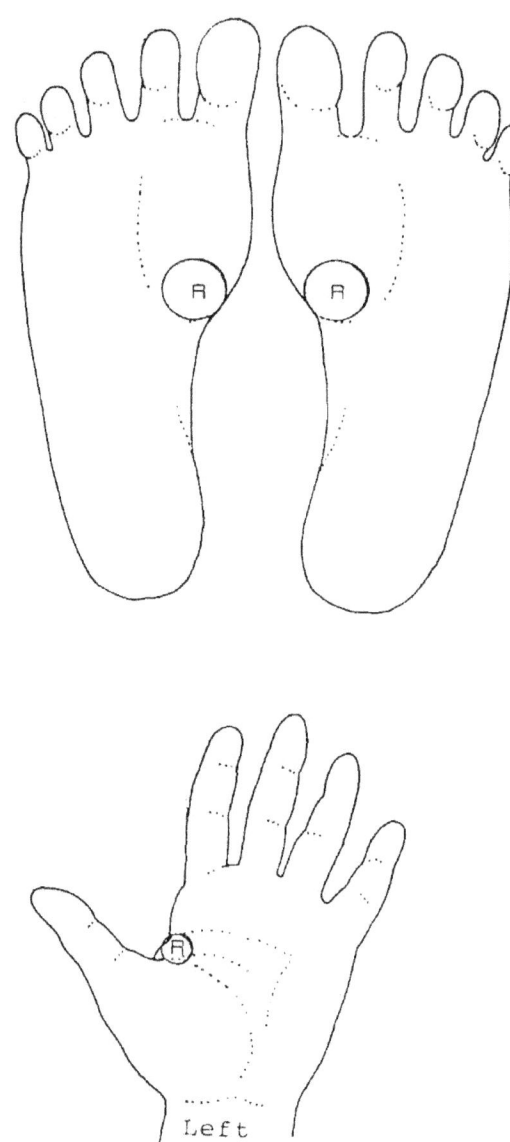

STOMACH MERIDIAN SYSTEM

Ileocecal Meridian System (d)

A. The ileocecal valve is located on the right side of the lower abdomen midway between the protruding pelvic bone and the naval.

B. An integral part of the digestive tract, the ileocecal valve is located between the small intestine and large intestine. From the stomach, food material enters the small intestine where essentially all digestion of nutrients, including vitamins, occurs. During this phase the ileocecal valve remains constricted. As digestion is completed here, the ileocecal valve relaxes and food material passes to the large intestine where there are no digestive enzymes produced, and water is absorbed.

C. In the weak Ileocecal Meridian System, the valve is either relaxed when it is supposed to be constricted or constricted when it is supposed to be relaxed. When this happens, undigested food is allowed to pass prematurely into an intestinal area where it can't get digested.

D. PROCEDURE

Locate reflex points 1 and 2 on the diagram on the following page. Point 1 is on the front of the right shoulder as you feel the top of your arm. Reflex point 2 is midway between the navel and the top of the hip bone that protrudes forward. While holding point 2 with the middle fingers of your right hand, grab your right shoulder with the left hand by wrapping your fingers around the shoulder, and pressing on reflex point 1 with the thumb. Press with the thumb using a rotary motion and about 4 lbs of pressure. Do this for 3 minutes.

Next move the left hand up the shoulder toward the neck and grab the muscle on top of the shoulder. While doing this, massage reflex point 2 with the right hand, using 4 lbs of pressure in a headward and footward motion. Do this for 3 minutes.

Perform this procedure every day (not with a full stomach) for two weeks. If discomfort occurs, during or after this process, discontinue the procedure.

Foods To Avoid - raw fruits and vegetables, salads, raw juices

<u>Foods To Include</u> - cooked rice, oatmeal, cooked vegetables, ripe bananas, bread, milk, lean well-cooked meat. Eat more frequent, small meals.

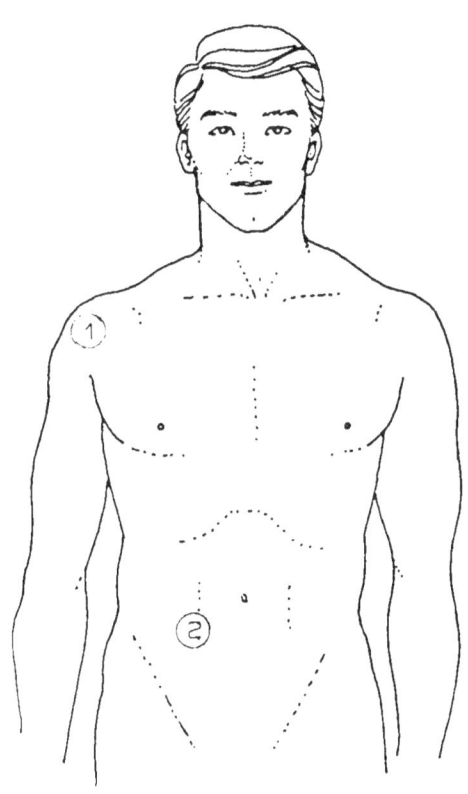

ILEOCECAL MERIDIAN SYSTEM

Intestine Meridian System (e)

A. The intestines snake throughout your abdomen.

B. The intestines are the major area of nutrient absorption. The intestines also assist in the breakdown of food matter.

C. A weak Intestines Meridian System will cause indigestion. This can result in many problems including excessive gas, weight gain, and lower abdominal cramping.

D. PROCEDURE

With one finger press into the abdomen, just above the navel, using about 5 lbs of pressure. Do this just below the navel as well. The more tender of these points is your reflex point #1 (usually above the navel).

Reflex point #2 is found on the right hand. Spread the fingers apart. Reflex point #2 is about 3/4 inches from the outside intersection of the thumb and forefinger in the fleshy part of the "V" formed there.

Place the right index finger and middle finger on reflex point #1. Grip the top of the right shoulder with the left hand and hold onto the muscle there. Now massage reflex point #1 for one minute. Next squeeze reflex point #2 with your left thumb and index finger, applying 3 to 5 lbs of pressure. Do this for 1 minute.

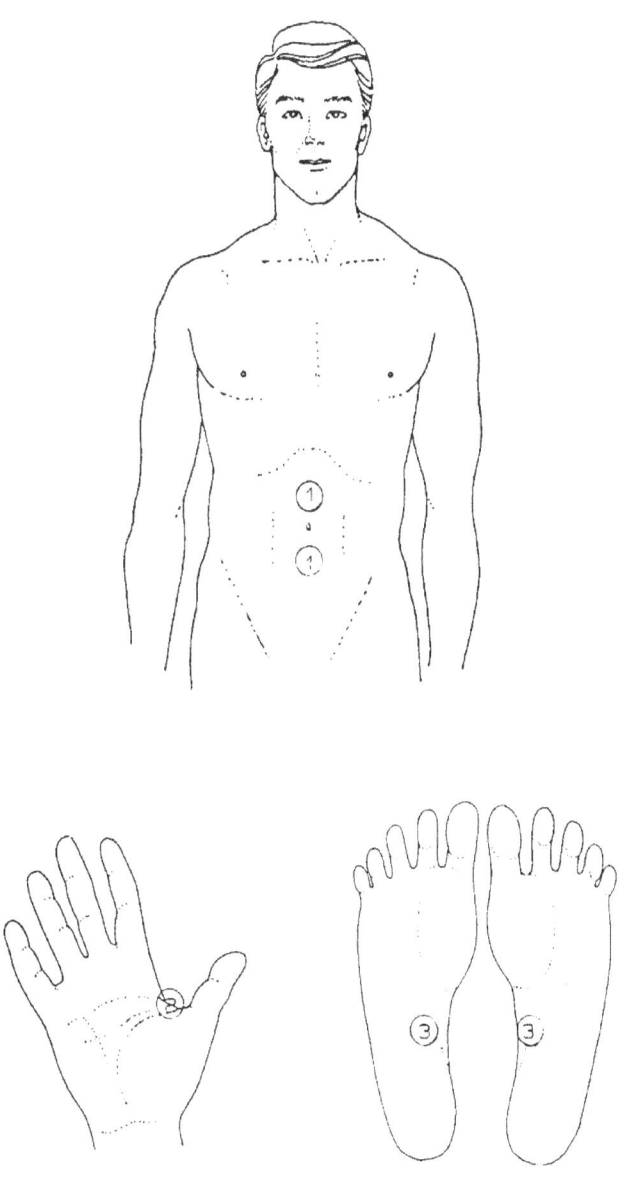

INTESTINE MERIDIAN SYSTEM

Next place your right hand on your right rib cage with the fingers aiming towards the body centerline. With the left hand, place the thumb one inch to the left of the navel and the index finger one inch to the right. Using about 3 lbs of pressure, press into the abdomen with both hands in the described position. As you do this, move the left hand upward and the right hand downward. Do not let the fingers slide on the skin, but move the tissue with the hand. You are stimulating the intestines. Do this 10 times, and coordinate it with respiration. Pressing into the abdomen on exhalation and relaxing the hold on inhalation.

Now massage reflex point #1 for one minute.

Reflex point #3 is a 2 square inch area on the bottom of each foot. Press your thumb into the center of this area, and apply moderate pressure (5 lbs) in a massaging fashion for 3 minutes. Be sure to do this to both feet.

This procedure should be performed every other day for one month. If discomfort occurs, during or after this process, discontinue the procedure.

Foods To Avoid - animal fats, sugar, too much raw fruit
Foods To Include - raw potatoes, pineapple

Kidney Meridian System (f)
A. Your kidneys are located behind your intestines in the back side of the lower abdomen.

B. The kidneys function to achieve a constant acid-base balance, and to maintain proper body water volume. They are essential organs involved in the electrical and chemical balance of your body as well as the excretory process.

C. Besides causing a lot of pain, malfunctioning kidneys can lower your resistance to infection by altering your normal acid-alkaline balance. Weak kidneys can increase blood pressure by making the heart pump harder to move body fluids, and affect skin tone and weight distribution. That aggravating 5 to 10 lbs that you can't seem to lose could be fluid retention if the kidney system enters into your health picture.

D. PROCEDURE

Trace with your finger one inch above the navel and four inches across to either side. Press in with 5 lbs of pressure using your index finger. Do this on both the right and left side of the abdomen. The more tender of the two is reflex #1. This reflex indicates which kidney is the weak one. Refer to the diagram.

There are two procedures for the Kidney Meridian System. Select only one of them to perform on yourself.

Procedure #1 - For those having frequent urination or uncomfortable urination.
Procedure #2 - For those having normal or infrequent urination without discomfort.

Procedure #1
If reflex #1 is on the right side of your body, place your left forefinger and middle finger there and exert a pressure of 5 lbs on this point. At the same time, place your right hand on the left shoulder grabbing the muscle on the top of the shoulder (reflex point # 2). Continue the 5 lbs pressure and the holding of the shoulder for 3 minutes.

If reflex #1 is on the left side of your body, reverse the hand position.

Find reflex point #4 on the bottom of each foot. Refer to the diagram on the following page. This point will be one inch toward your toes from the center of your arch, and one inch from the inside edge of the foot. Massage reflex point #4 for 3 minutes on each foot. Take long slow inhalations, and short forceful exhalations while you do this.

This procedure should be performed everyday for 2 weeks. If discomfort occurs, during or after this process, discontinue the procedure.

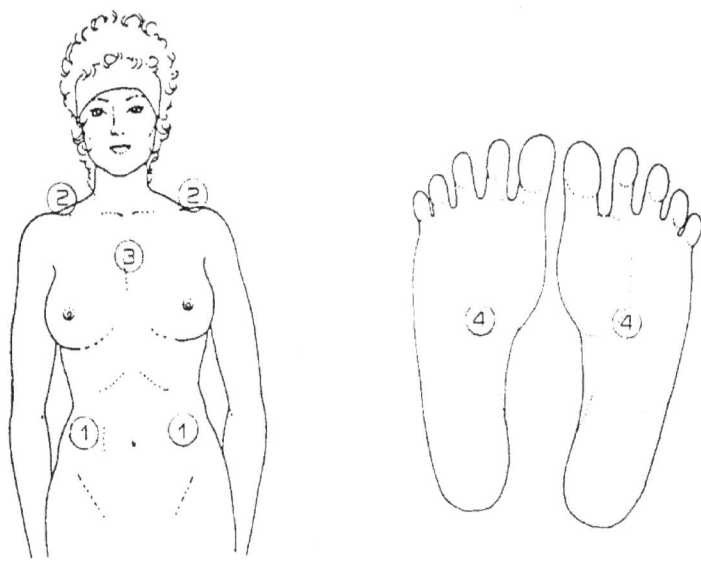

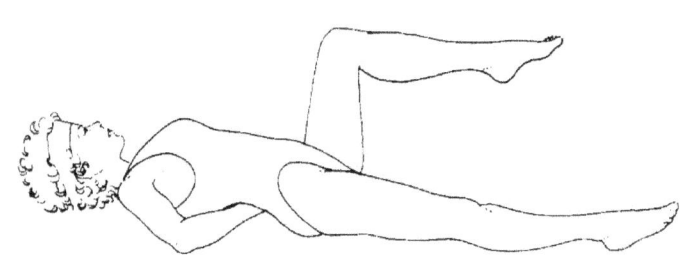

KIDNEY MERIDIAN SYSTEM

Procedure #2

Find reflex point #3 on the sternum (center of chest). This point should be tender to touch (about 3 lbs of pressure) so move your finger up or down the sternum until you locate the tender reflex. Using 3 lbs of pressure, massage reflex points 1 and 3, simultaneously. Continue for 3 minutes.

Next place your hand directly under reflex point #1 palm down, fingers against your back. Refer to the diagram on the previous page. Raise your leg on the side of reflex point #1 with bent knee as you inhale. Now as you exhale, straighten your leg, lower it slowly to the floor, and press with your hand into your back and headward. Repeat this movement for three inhalations and three exhalations. Now bring your arms to your side and relax.

Find reflex point #4 on the bottom of each foot. Refer to the diagram on the previous page. This point will be one inch toward your toes from the center of your arch, and one inch from the inside edge of the foot. Massage reflex point #4 for 3 minutes on each foot. Take long slow inhalations, and short forceful exhalations while you do this.

This procedure should be performed everyday for 2 weeks. If discomfort occurs, during or after this process, discontinue the procedure.

Foods To Avoid - salt, red meat, alcoholic beverages, coffee, cigarettes, black or green tea.
Foods To Include - fresh vegetables, 12 glasses of pure water per day

Liver Meridian System (g)

A. The liver is located in the upper right quadrant of the abdomen. It extends from just above your navel to several inches under your rib cage.

B. The liver is a fairly large and important gland. It is the major organ of detoxification in your body. It is an essential organ.

C. When your liver is weak, the quality of your blood is affected. Recurring illnesses, lack of energy, foggy thinking, and varicose veins are a few of the companions of this system.

D. PROCEDURE

Place your left hand over your sternum (center of chest) palm down, so that your index finger lies just under your collar bone. With fingers close together, bend fingers slightly so that you can press their tips into your chest on the right side. Reflex point #1 is underneath your 4th finger, and should be a little tender to about 3 lbs of pressure.

Reflex point #2 is 3 inches to the right of the navel and 2 inches down.

Massage point #1 with the index and middle finger of your left hand for 1 minute using 3 lbs of pressure.

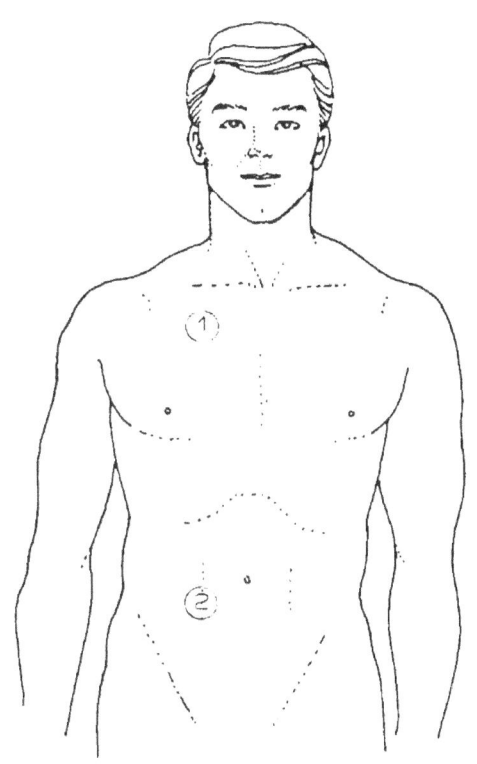

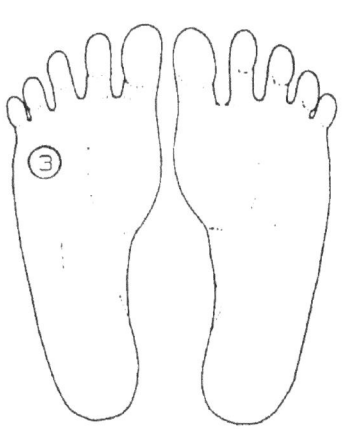

LIVER MERIDIAN SYSTEM

Now with your left hand still on point #1, locate point #2 and massage with the index and middle finger of the right hand using 3 lbs of pressure for 3 minutes.

Next, place your left hand on your stomach with the palm on the navel and your right hand on your right rib cage so that your little finger is resting on the last rib.

As you exhale, your left hand presses into the body and upward. At the same time, the right hand presses into the body and towards the left side. Relax the hands on inhalation, and repeat the pressure on the next exhalation. Do this for five breathing cycles.

Now relax and breathe normally for 2 minutes.

Reflex point #3 is on the bottom of the right foot 1 1/2 inches below the 4th toe. Massage this point with the left thumb for 3 minutes with 5 lbs of pressure while breathing slowly and deeply.

Do this procedure everyday for 3 weeks. If discomfort occurs, during or after this process, discontinue the procedure.

Foods To Avoid - alcoholic beverages, coffee, tea, cigarettes
Foods To Include - fresh vegetables, especially green and yellow ones

Pancreas Meridian System (h)

A. The pancreas is located in the center of the chest just below the sternum (breastbone). It is almost horizontal in position, angling slightly towards the front.

B. The pancreas secretes enzymes into the beginning of the intestines to assist in breaking down proteins, fats, and carbohydrates for absorption by the intestinal walls. The pancreas also affects the secretion of natural insulin in the body.

C. A weakness of the pancreas will result in digestive disturbances and weight gain or loss due to fat digestion. Unstable energy levels will also result from improper blood sugar levels.

D. PROCEDURE

Refer to diagrams on the following page for reflex point locations. Locate reflex point #1. It is in the fleshy part of the right hand that is the bottom of the thumb. Reflex point #2 is directly under the sternum (breastbone) above the stomach. Reflex point #3 is on top of the lowest rib in the center of the left rib cage. Reflex point #4 is underneath the lowest rib in the center of the right rib cage. Place the left thumb on reflex point #1. With the left hand fingers on the back of the right hand, massage reflex point #1 with the left thumb using 3 lbs of pressure for 1 minute.

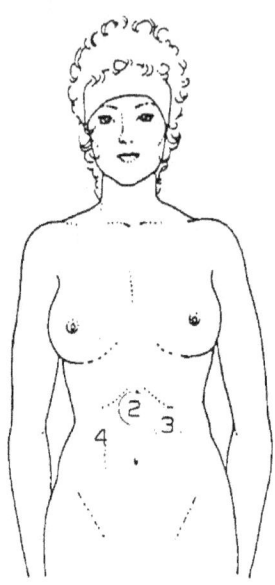

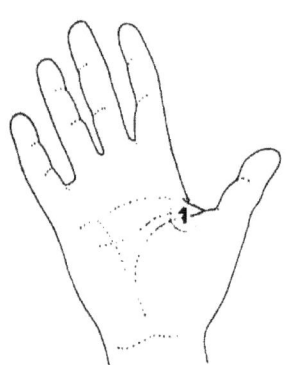

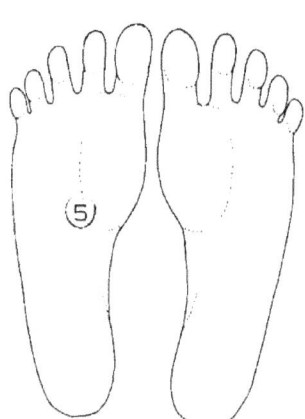

PANCREAS MERIDIAN SYSTEM

Next, stop massaging, but keep the 3 lbs of pressure on reflex point #1 with the left thumb. At the same time, place the index and middle fingers of the right hand on reflex point #2. Exert 3 lbs of pressure for 1 minute.

Now continue the left thumb pressure on reflex point #1 and move your hands to reflex point #3. Press on this point with the index and middle fingers of the right hand using 3 lbs of pressure for 1 minute.

While continuing your hold on reflex point #1, move the right index and middle finger to reflex point #4 so that the fingers curl up under the right rib cage exerting approximately 3 lbs of pressure for 1 minute.

Now relax the right arm by resting it at your side. With the index and middle fingers of your left hand, massage reflex point #2 with very light pressure for 3 minutes.

Reflex point #5 is on the bottom of the right foot at the top of the arch just below the 2nd and 3rd toe. Massage this point with the left thumb for 3 minutes while breathing more deeply than you normally do.

Let both arms fall to your sides, and relax for several minutes before getting up.

This procedure should be done every other day for 2 weeks. If discomfort occurs, during or after this process, discontinue the procedure.

Foods To Avoid - sugar, alcoholic beverages, carbohydrates
Foods To Include - raw cabbage, high protein foods

Prostate Meridian System (i)
A. The prostate gland is located just below the bladder.

B. The prostate gland produces nutrient-rich secretions which add to the population of sperm as they pass through the prostatic urethra.

C. Weakness of the prostate may cause sexual dysfunction, lack of sex drive, and infertility.

D. PROCEDURE

Refer to the diagram on the next for reflex point location.

Reflex point #1 is midway between the scrotum and the anus. Press this point with one finger. It may or may not be tender in the Prostate Meridian System. Hold 3 lbs of pressure here for 1 minute. Reflex point #2 is at the centerline of the body just above the pubic bone. Reflex point #3 is the muscle mass on top of the right shoulder.

With the left hand grab Reflex point #3. Hold firmly while contacting reflex point #2 with the right hand. Massage reflex point #2 with 3 lbs of pressure for 3 minutes while holding reflex point #3.

With your thumb, apply 5 lbs of pressure to the back of the foot just below the level of the ankle. Do this for 3 minutes on each foot.

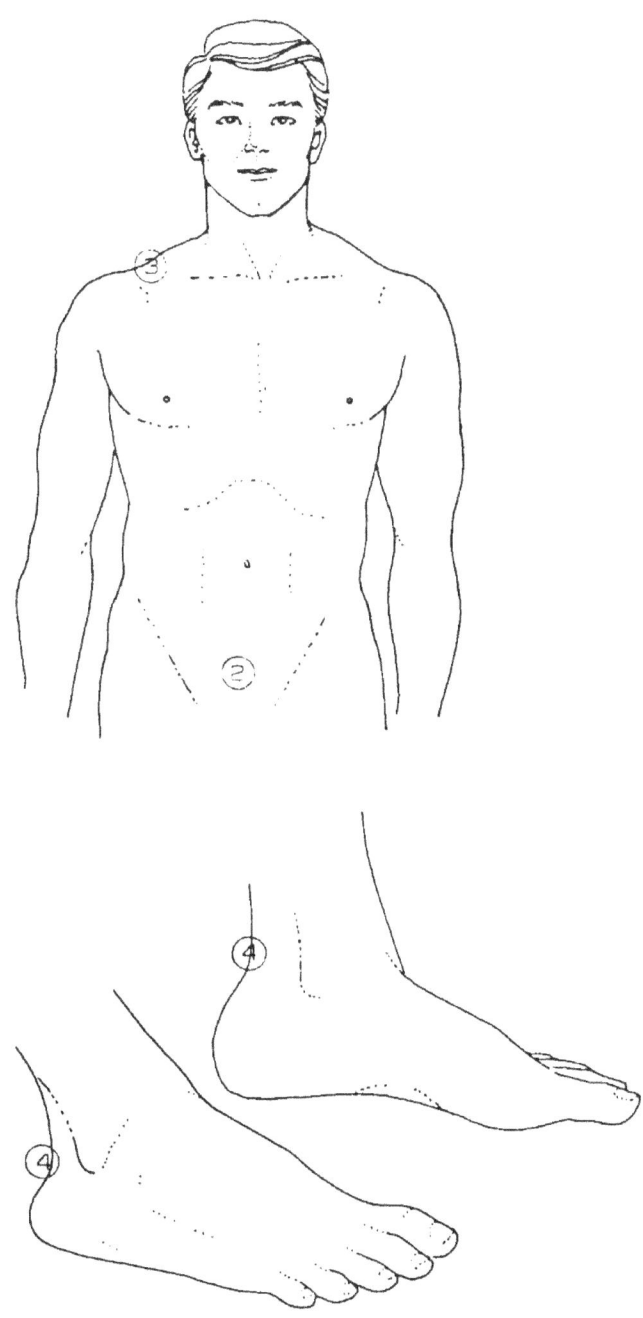

PROSTATE MERIDIAN SYSTEM

This procedure should be done every other day, for 3 months. If discomfort occurs, during or after this process, discontinue the procedure.

Foods To Avoid - alcoholic beverages, cigarettes, white bread
Foods To Include - dairy products, wheat germ, whole wheat breads, pumpkin seeds.

EXERCISE FOR THE PROSTATE

Lie down on your back. With bent knees, try to press the bottoms of your feet together. Let your hips relax, so that your knees fall to each side towards the floor.

In this position, raise your legs up and then down, continuously pressing the feet together, isometrically. Start doing this for 30 seconds per day, and gradually increase to 3 minutes per day.

Respiratory Meridian System (j)

A. We are primarily concerned with the two lungs occupying the chest cavity, but the throat and sinuses are affected also in this system.

B. The lungs are responsible for getting oxygen into the blood, and removing carbon dioxide from the blood.

C. Weakness in the lung function will lead to repeated respiratory distress, susceptibility to colds and flu, allergies, and asthmatic conditions.

D. PROCEDURE

Run the index finger of both hands along the bottom of the jaw to where it turns up toward the ears. Press into the neck at these points simultaneously with 3 lbs of pressure. Now maintain this pressure while pulling the fingers down the neck as they naturally follow the deep grooves on either side. Do this 6 or 8 times starting just under the ear and pulling down.

Refer to the diagrams in this section, when locating the following reflex points.

Reflex point #1 is just under the collarbone (clavicle), 1 inch inward from the nipple line.

Reflex point #2 is just below reflex point #1 between the next two ribs.

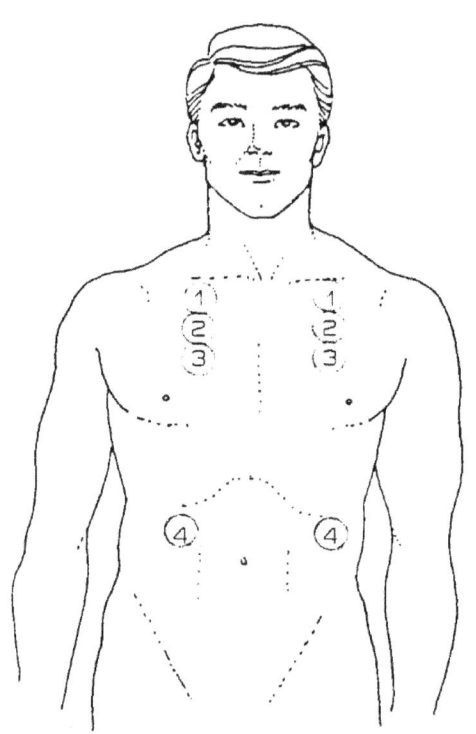

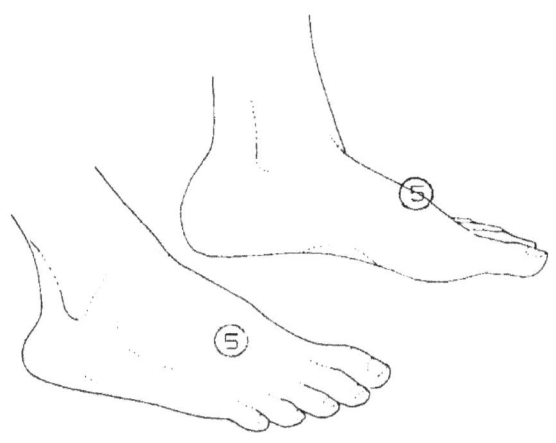

RESPIRATORY MERIDIAN SYSTEM

Reflex point #3 is just below reflex point #2 between the <u>next</u> two ribs.

Check all six of these points for tenderness. Gently massage any of these reflexes that are tender with light pressure until the tenderness goes away.

With the four fingers of both hands, press under the rib cage on both sides with about 3 lbs of pressure. Massage this area by moving the fingers from side to side so that the hands move away from each other, and then towards each other. Do this for 1 minute.

Reflex #4 is straight down from the nipple line at the bottom of the rib cage. With the index and middle finger of the right hand, massage these points for 2 minutes each.

Reflex point #5 is on the top of both feet in the middle of the foot, one inch from the base of the toes. With very light pressure (1 lb) massage this area on both feet using the opposite thumb. (right thumb massages left foot, and vice versa) Do this for 2 minutes per foot while breathing slowly and deeply.

This procedure should be done every other day for 2 months. If discomfort occurs, during or after this process, discontinue the procedure.

<u>Foods To Avoid</u> - dairy products (with the possible exception of yogurt) alcoholic beverages cigarettes, pipes, cigars sugar wheat flour
<u>Foods To Include</u> - radishes, carrots

Uterus Meridian System (k)
THIS SYNDROME APPLIES ONLY TO WOMEN WHO ARE NOT PREGNANT.

A. The uterus if located immediately above the bladder and the vagina.

B. The main purpose of the uterus is to serve as a site for implantation and nourishment of a new embryo, after the freshly fertilized ovum is conducted through the uterine tubes from the ovary. If the ovum is unfertilized, the uterus then has the job of sloughing off the ovum in the monthly menses.

C. A weak uterus can be responsible for infertility from failure to provide a fertile implantation site. A weak uterus can also result in menstrual irregularities, lack of sexual desire, cramping during menses, painful inter- course, and many general aches and pains.

D. PROCEDURE

Refer to the diagram on the following page for reflex point location.

Reflex point #1 is on top of the right shoulder.

Reflex point #2 is on the sternum (breastbone). This point will vary in location from woman to woman. Move your fingers up and down the sternum until you find a tender spot. It should be near the center.

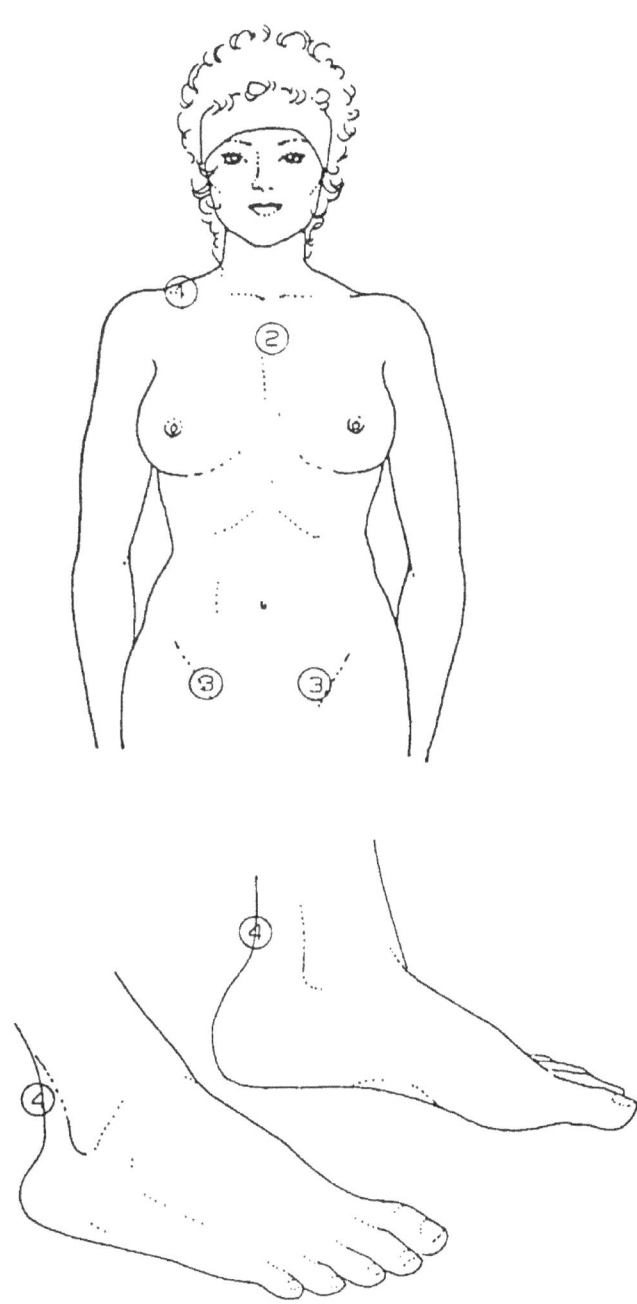

UTERUS MERIDIAN SYSTEM

Reflex point #3 is along the inguinal ligament, or the indentation in the skin where the leg meets the lower abdomen. Again, the location of this point will vary from woman to woman, but will always lie along this inguinal ligament line and may be on the right or left side of the body. You may find more than one reflex point in this area depending on the severity of the problem. Choose the most tender point as your reflex point #3.

With your left hand contact reflex point #1, and hold the muscles there. Now massage reflex point #3 with about 3 lbs of pressure using the index and middle fingers of the right hand. Do this for 3 minutes while holding reflex point #1.

Next, with your right hand still on reflex point #3 and exerting 3 lbs of pressure, contact reflex point #2 with your left index and middle fingers and massage gently (1 lb pressure) for 3 minutes.

With your thumb, apply 5 lbs of pressure to the back of the foot just below the level of the ankle. Do this for 3 minutes on each foot.

This procedure should be performed every day for 2 months. If discomfort occurs, during or after this process, discontinue the procedure.

Foods To Avoid - alcoholic beverages
Foods To Include - seafood, seaweeds, yogurt

Adrenal Meridian System (m)

A. The adrenal glands are located on top of the kidneys, one on each side of the body.

B. The adrenal glands are part of the endocrine system. They are responsible for the secretion of biochemicals and hormones which play a role in the metabolism of protein, carbohydrates, electrolytes, and water. They also produce biochemicals which allow you to deal with stress.

C. If your adrenal glands are weak, you are likely to handle stress very poorly. Weak adrenal glands will frequently cause sexual dysfunction, and high or low blood pressure.

D. PROCEDURE

Refer to the diagrams on the following page for reflex point location.

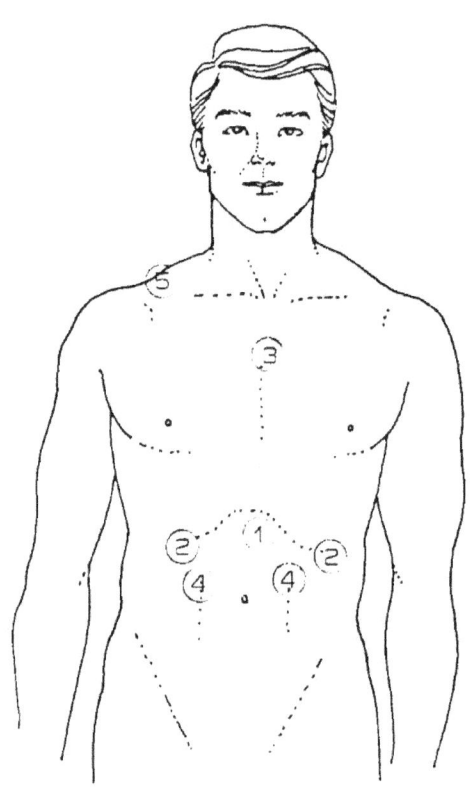

ADRENAL MERIDIAN SYSTEM

Place your hands above your abdomen with the palms against your ribs, so that the ends of your middle fingers touch one another. Now arch your hands, maintaining contact with the finger tips, so that the fingers of both hands are pressed back to back. Allow the fingers to press into the chest area between the ribs (reflex point #1), just under the sternum (breastbone). Now place your thumbs 6 to 8 inches apart, and 1 inch above the bottom of the ribs. Your thumbs are now on reflex points #2.

With a slightly bouncing motion, alternately press in with the thumbs and the fingers both sides at the same time. You will press with the thumbs, then as you lift the thumbs, press with the fingers, then lift the fingers, and press with the thumbs.

IF YOU HAVE HIGH BLOOD PRESSURE, THIS SHOULD BE DONE VERY SLOWLY——ONE CYCLE PER SECOND FOR 1O SECONDS.

IF YOU HAVE NORMAL OR LOW BLOOD PRESSURE, DO THIS MORE RAPIDLY——TWO CYCLES PER SECOND FOR 1O SECONDS.

Reflex point #3 is located in the middle of the sternum.

Reflex points #4 are one inch above the navel, and two inches to either side. Apply 3 lbs of pressure with the right index and middle finger to reflex points #4 for 1 minute each. At the same time, lightly massage reflex point #3 with the left index and middle finger.

Now grab reflex point #5 on top of the right shoulder with your left hand. Keep a grasp on reflex point #5 while massaging reflex points #4 with the right index and middle finger for 3 minutes each. Use light pressure of 1-2 lbs.

This procedure should be done every other day for one month. If discomfort occurs, during or after this process, discontinue the procedure.

Foods To Avoid - coffee, black or green tea
Foods To Include - rice, whole grains, nuts, and seeds

Cardiovascular Meridian System (n)

A. The heart is located between the breasts slightly to the left of center of the body.

B. The heart is a muscle which continuously pumps blood throughout the body via the cardiovascular system. Its pumping rate speeds up or slows down in response to the body tissues needs for oxygen laden blood.

C. Weakness of the myocardium can cause improper rate or strength in this pumping motion resulting in inadequate blood/oxygen supply to the body tissues.

D. PROCEDURE

Grasp both rib cages with your hands so that your fingers are tucked under the last rib. As you inhale pull headward with your hands, exerting an upward pressure on the ribs of about 3 lbs. (If this is uncomfortable, you are doing it too hard.) As you inhale and pull up on the ribs, raise your right leg keeping it straight at the knee. If you are left handed, raise the left leg, instead of the right. Do this for 3 breathing cycles.

Now do this for 3 more breathing cycles, raising the opposite leg.

Reflex point #1 is 4 inches down from the center of the collarbone on the left side. Refer to the diagram on the following page to locate reflex points.

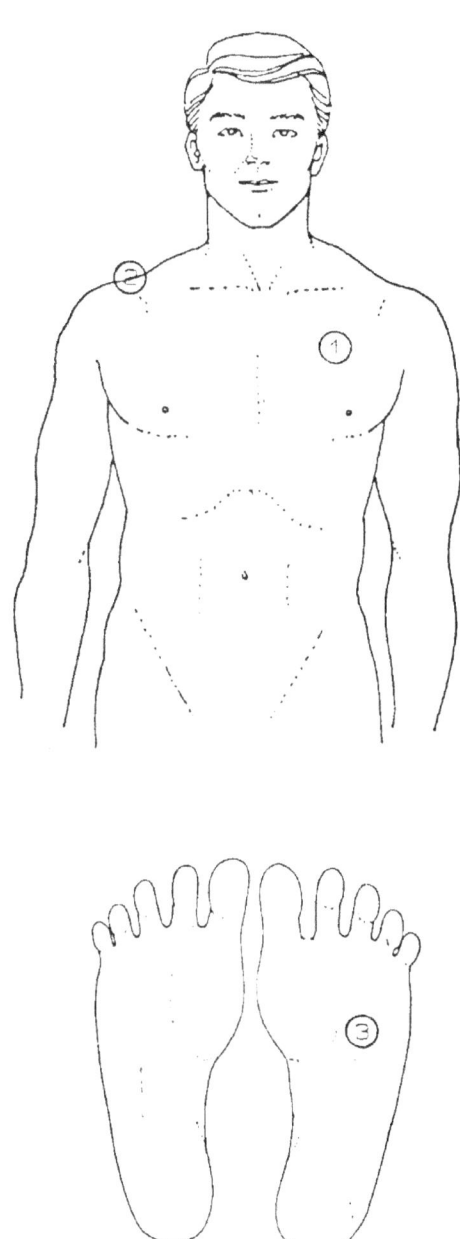

CARDIOVASCULAR MERIDIAN SYSTEM

Reflex point #2 is the musculature making up the top of the right shoulder.

Grasp reflex point #2 with the left hand while massaging reflex point #1 with 3 lbs of pressure for 3 minutes using the right index and middle fingers.

Reflex point #3 is located on the bottom of the left foot at the top of the arch, directly down from the middle toe. Using the right thumb, massage this point with 5 lbs of pressure for 3 minutes.

This procedure should be performed every day for 2 weeks. If discomfort occurs, during or after this process, discontinue the procedure.

<u>Foods To Avoid</u> - salt, fats, fried foods, pork, cholesterol foods
<u>Foods To Include</u> - fresh vegetables, safflower oil for cooking and salads

Acknowledgments

I am extremely grateful to two pioneers of alternative health care. Many of the techniques that they developed became the foundation of *Internal Fitness*.

Major Bertrand De Jarnette, D.C. developed Chiropractic Manipulative Reflex Technique as part of Sacro Occipital Technique.

George J. Goodheart, D.C. advanced the development of Applied Kinesiology.

In addition, I would like to thank the following people for helping me with this project:

Jean A. Cammareri for her illustrations and cover design.

Anne Basto, my wife, for her loving support and encouragement in the writing of this book. Anne has completed a terrific adventure novel that should be available on Amazon.com by the end of 2013. Look for *Fast Lane to Sunset*. You won't be disappointed.